CAROL VORDERMAN'S
EAT TO BEAT
CELLULITE
RECIPES

WITH ANITA BEAN

D1347026

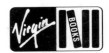

CHECK WITH YOUR DOCTOR

Before starting any diet programme, you should consult your doctor. In particular, this should be done with regard to any allergies you may have to the foods or drinks recommended or contained within these recipes. The recipes may not be suitable for everyone. Pregnant women should be especially careful and ensure that their doctor advises that the recipes are suitable for them. If you are taking medication or have any medical condition, you should check with your doctor first.

While the authors have made every effort to ensure that the information contained in this book is as accurate as possible, it is advisory only and should not be used as an alternative to seeking specialist medical advice. The authors and publisher cannot be held responsible for actions that may be taken by a reader as a result of reliance on the information contained in this book, which are taken entirely at the reader's own risk.

Carol Vorderman was assisted in the writing of this book by:

Anita Bean BSc, an award-winning nutritionist and the author of 15 books, including *Carol Vorderman's Detox for Life* series and, as co-author, of *Carol Vorderman's 30-Day Cellulite Plan*. She writes for numerous magazines and newspapers and is also a broadcaster on TV and radio.

First published in Great Britain in 2006 by
Virgin Books Ltd, Thames Wharf Studios, Rainville Road, London W6 9HA

A catalogue record for this book is available from the British Library

ISBN 07535 1067 7

All photography by David Loftus
Designed and typeset by Smith & Gilmour, London

Printed and bound in Great Britain by Bath Press

Contents

INTRODUCTION

Ever since I first became involved with the 'detox' way of eating, I have been asked countless times about health and beauty products and superfoods and particular fad diets.

One of the issues which crops up time after time is cellulite, particularly for women over the age of 30. In the *30-Day Cellulite Plan* published in 2004, we put together a complete plan that includes food, exercise and treatments and creams. Using the plan a number of volunteers bravely agreed to have photographs taken before and after their 30 days. The results were astonishing. Their 'orange peel' seemed to have burned off. Dimples had disappeared and the heavy look that legs can somehow gain had been replaced by a far sleeker image. Not only that, the skin all over their bodies had changed, losing the beginnings of a crepey look. They felt fitter and had more energy than they'd had for years.

And they are not alone. As the years continue to roll by and birthdays pass by in the night, the issues of weight and how your body looks occupies more and more time. Even the skinny minxes have their problems (thank goodness). Be honest, how many times have you stood in front of the mirror and wished that you could just drag all the skin and flesh upwards? Or suffered the misery of a changing room with lights shining directly down on your body, imitating the sun at high noon and showing up every ripple of flesh in the most unflattering light possible. Ugh! I'll never understand why shops continue to light their dressing rooms so badly because we'll never buy the clothes that way!

Anyway, after the success of the original Cellulite Plan, we were contacted by many women who now enjoy a cellulite-free body and who wanted more recipes to encourage them to continue with their plan. That is how this book was born.

In *Eat to Beat Cellulite* we've put together nearly 100 recipes with plenty of nutritional notes giving you the calorific content, fat content, health statistics and much much more. I have to say the food looks and tastes fabulous and believe me, if I can cook these dishes, anybody can. The days of Grade C in cookery lessons are long since behind me, but with these recipes I can turn out meals that everyone is happy with, especially me. Ha.

We've also included lists of superfoods and explained why they can help directly with reducing your bumps and ridges. Did you know for instance that mango helps to protect you against the sun's rays and improves your appetite control? Or that broccoli can help to strengthen bones? Oranges strengthen collagen in the skin's layers and tomatoes help to combat wrinkles. Marvellous isn't it? Turn these gorgeous foods into 'Blueberry Muffins with Apple Spread' or 'Dahl with Sweet Potatoes and Coconut' and you'll think you're cheating, but you won't be.

That's why I'm delighted with *Eat to Beat Cellulite*.

We have recipes to suit all palates and all times of the day from a fabulous granola for breakfast to pilaff for lunch or supper. I hope you enjoy these dishes as much as we have and that you'll be prancing around in your bikini by the next time you go on holiday.

All the best.

Carol Vorderman

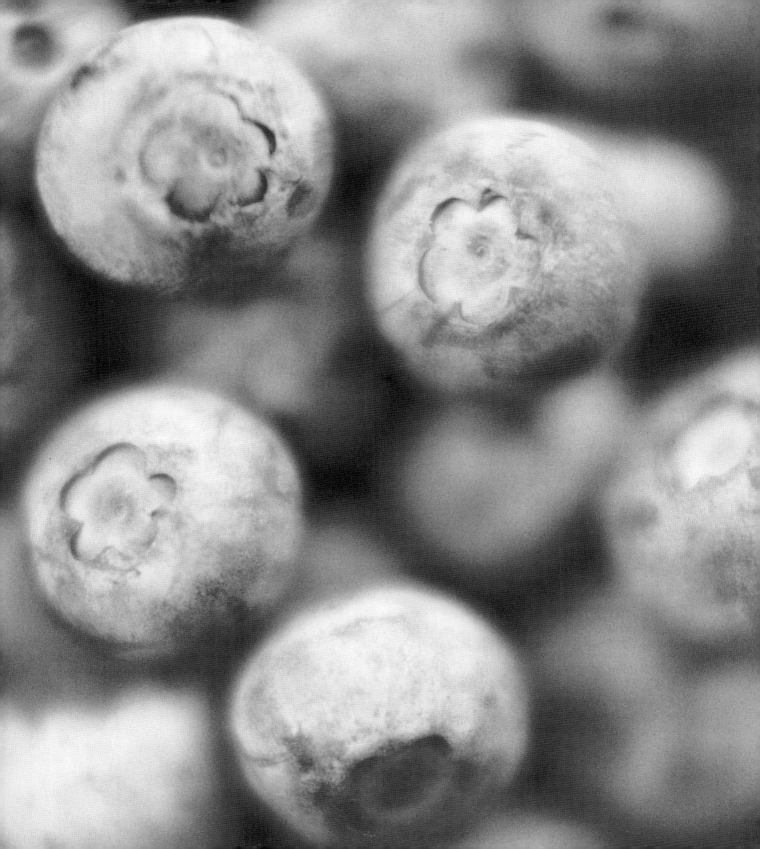

CHAPTER 1
HOW TO
BEAT
CELLULITE

Many of you picking up this book may have already read the *30-Day Cellulite Plan* and so know all about the causes of cellulite, but for those of you who need a little reminder and particularly for those who have bought this book with a view to tackling those dimples for the first time and have not read the Plan, here's a little reminder of what it's all about.

Cellulite is the name given to the lumpy, dimply fat that's stored under your skin and we're all susceptible as we get older – even slim people. It appears most commonly around the hips and thighs. But this orange-peel skin can also occur on the stomach and upper arms. It plagues around 95 per cent of women over the age of 25, but many under 25 can also have it to some degree. It can feel spongy and soft, or it can feel hard and cold. It's baffled doctors for decades and there have been all sorts of speculations about what causes it.

What is cellulite?

Cellulite is comprised of fat and fluids trapped in pockets of connective tissue underneath the skin. It is more common in women because, in addition to carrying more fat on their thighs and buttocks, the collagen support structure around fat cells is weaker in women than it is in men, sometimes causing the cells to pucker. The thin layer of connective tissue between fat cells starts to thicken and pull together around the fat, causing the tiny dimples and irregularities characteristic of cellulite. The fat inside the cells bulges out and the more fat you have, the worse the bulging.

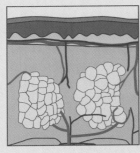 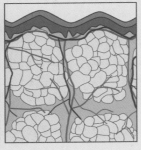

1. Normal fat deposits are shown lying underneath relatively smooth skin.

2. Excessive fat cells stretch the tissue between them and push out underneath the skin causing bulges.

What causes it?

There are an awful lot of theories about the causes of cellulite – most of which are unproven – but cellulite tends to run in families, suggesting an hereditary link. If your mother had cellulite, you've probably inherited the genes that favour fat storage around the hips and thighs as well as weaker collagen, both of which contribute to cellulite formation.

The fat–muscle connection

Looking at the scientific evidence, cellulite is essentially the result of two things: too much fat and too little muscle. Simply put, when the underlying muscle becomes too thin and the overlying fat becomes too thick, there is no firm base for the skin, which then takes on the wobbly, irregular appearance we call cellulite. This explains why even slim – or 'under-muscled' – women get it.

If you don't use it, you lose it

Failing to take enough exercise has serious consequences. Without regular toning exercise, you start to lose muscle after the age of about 20. Between the ages of 20 and 30 years, the average, non-exercising woman loses about 2 kg (5 lb), a further 2 kg (5 lb) between 30 and 40 years and a similar amount each decade thereafter. The result is a loss of strength as well as an increase in fat storage.

The metabolic slow-down

As you lose muscle, your metabolic rate drops (the number of calories you burn daily to maintain essential body functions). Muscle is calorie-burning tissue, so the less you have, the fewer calories you need. So, as you get older you need fewer calories just to maintain your body weight. For every 2-kg loss of muscle, your metabolic rate drops by 5 per cent.

Why you get fatter with age

This age-related muscle loss means that you burn fewer calories and store more of them as fat. Even if you continue eating the same amount of food and keeping the same lifestyle, your weight will increase as your body converts the excess calories into stored fat. It's a gradual process, of course, but can result in a gain of 7 kg (15 lb) of fat each decade.

It all goes in the wrong direction!

But there's worse news. While you're losing muscle and gaining fat, the scales may not give you the whole picture. They may show only a 5-kg (10-lb) weight gain but, in fact, you've gained 7 kg (15 lb) of *fat*. You've also lost 2 kg (5 lb) of muscle, so you've got a 9-kg (20-lb) change in body composition – all in the wrong direction!

The body fat crisis

So, let's do the maths. By the age of 50 years – i.e. over three decades – you could have lost 6 kg (13 lb) of muscle and gained 21 kg (46 lb) of fat. That's a body composition change of 27 kg (59 lb) and a weight gain (according to the scales) of 15 kg (33 lb). But, by now, you could be carrying almost half (50 per cent) of your body fat as fat!

It all ends in the wobble

Where's this fat going to go? For most women, it will be stored around the hips and thighs. But the problem is that there is no longer a firm foundation for the network of connective tissue that holds the skin to the muscle. When an area has too much fat, too little muscle and weak connective tissue, it loses its normal firm appearance and takes on the characteristic wobbly appearance of cellulite.

How to eat to beat cellulite

No one has ever claimed that getting rid of cellulite is easy. Just as it takes years to develop, so it can't be eradicated overnight. There are literally hundreds of cellulite 'cures' ranging from diets and pills to creams and salon treatments. In the *30-day Cellulite Plan* (Virgin Books), we tested many treatments on a group of volunteers to find out what worked and what didn't.

After 30 days, the most effective method for reducing cellulite was a combination of sensible dieting and exercise. Those women who followed either the diet alone or the exercise plan alone got noticeable improvements, but those who did both got the best results. On average, the women following the diet and exercise plan (with or without creams and beauty treatments) lost around 4 kg (9 lb) in 30 days and, as their 'before' and 'after' photos show, there was a dramatic improvement in the appearance of their cellulite.

> Reducing your calorie intake while increasing your daily calorie burn creates a calorie deficit, so your body has no choice but to use up its fat stores.

Forget fad diets

Many people make the mistake of following the latest diet fad, which is a recipe for disaster. Drastic calorie chopping can make you lethargic and weak, leading to your body actually hoarding rather than burning fat, slow down your metabolic rate and cause you to burn muscle as fuel. Yo-yo dieting can make you fatter because you lose muscle and gain fat with each diet-cycle. And a study in the *Journal of the American Dietetic Association* suggests that failing to stick to a diet not only confuses your metabolism but also lowers your confidence and self-esteem. With a sensible healthy eating and exercise plan, though, you can lose fat (not muscle), improve your health and get fitter.

Experts agree that between ¹/₂ kg (1 lb) and 1 kg (2 lb) is a healthy and effective rate of weight loss. And ¹/₂ kg of fat equates to roughly 3500 calories. So to lose ¹/₂ kg in a week you need to burn 3500 more calories than you take in. This isn't as daunting as it sounds: lose 300 calories a day by foregoing two biscuits and drinking one less glass of wine and step up your expenditure by 200 calories a day and you'll lose ¹/₂ kg a week.

EIGHT GUIDELINES TO BEAT CELLULITE

- Eat five or more portions of fruit and vegetables each day
- Avoid saturated and processed (hydrogenated) fats
- Eat foods high in fibre and water
- Include low GI grains and cereals in your daily diet
- Eat more beans and lentils
- Eat nuts and seeds regularly
- Drink at least 6–8 glasses (1¹/₂ litres) of water daily
- Avoid refined sugars and flour; salt and artificial additives

THE GI EXPLAINED

The GI is simply a measure of how the body reacts to foods containing carbohydrate. High GI foods are digested more rapidly and cause a rapid surge in blood sugar level. They have a GI number above 70 (glucose has the highest score at 100). Those with a low GI number – below 55 – are digested more slowly and produce a slower and smaller rise in your blood sugar. And those in between 55 and 70 are classed as medium GI.

Satisfy your hunger

The key to losing excess weight and cellulite is to choose foods that are nutritious, enjoyable and make you feel satisfied. If you simply limit calories you'll feel hungry and deprived and sooner or later will regain the weight. You need to make food choices that help you feel full with fewer calories. This is why low GI eating works.

There is concrete scientific evidence that a low GI diet helps people lose more weight than standard low-fat diets. What's more, people are more likely to maintain their weight loss in the long term.

LOW GI EATING

Think of low GI eating as a healthy, balanced eating plan rather than a weight-loss regime. It focuses on fruit, vegetables, wholegrains, low-fat protein foods, nuts, beans and lentils. The idea with low GI eating is to eat slow-burning food regularly throughout the day. This produces a steady level of sugar in the bloodstream, which means that you will be full of energy rather than suffering tiredness. But there are lots of health benefits, too, from improving your concentration to cutting the risks of high blood pressure, diabetes and heart disease.

LOW GI EATING CAN HELP YOU LOSE WEIGHT BECAUSE:

▸ Low GI foods are more filling and keep you satisfied longer than high GI foods
▸ Low GI foods help to control your hunger and appetite naturally
▸ Low GI foods keep insulin levels low, which helps you to burn more fat and less muscle.

	LOW GI	MEDIUM GI	HIGH GI
Biscuits		Digestive biscuits	Most biscuits
Bread and cakes	Breads containing oats, soy, cracked wheat and seeds Coarse grain bread Rye bread Stoneground wholemeal bread	Chapatti Oatcakes Pitta bread Rye crispread	Bagels Crackers Doughnuts French bread sticks Gluten-free bread Regular sliced wholemeal Rice cakes White bread and rolls
Dairy Products	Low-fat dairy products, e.g. milk and yoghurt, soya milk	Ice cream	
Fish	All types		
Fruit	Most fresh fruit, e.g. apples, apricots, bananas, grapes, kiwi fruit, mango oranges, strawberries Most fruit juice	Dried figs Pineapple Raisins Sultanas Tinned fruit	
Grains and cereals	Barley Bulgar wheat Cous cous Muesli Porridge Oatmeal	Muesli bars	Most breakfast cereals, e.g. cornflakes, rice crispies, bran flakes Breakfast bars
Meat	All kinds of poultry and lean cuts of meat		
Nuts and seeds	All kinds		
Pasta, Noodles & Rice	All kinds (see High GI)	Basmati rice Rice noodles Wholegrain (brown) rice	Gluten-free pasta White rice
Pulses and Vegetables	Beans Chickpeas Lentils Most vegetables, e.g. cucumber, broccoli, except potatoes Sweet potatoes Sweetcorn Yams		Baked, boiled, chipped or mashed potatoes
Spreads, Sweets & Sugar	Honey	Jam	Soft drinks All sweets Sugar

HOW LOW GI EATING WORKS

High-fibre foods, such as beans, lentils, oats, fruit and vegetables release their energy slowly, so they have a low GI. Simply put: foods with a low GI tend to make you feel satisfied for longer and less inclined to snack on unhealthy foods. Protein-rich foods – meat, fish, chicken and eggs – and pure fats – oils, butter and margarine – contain no carbohydrate so these foods are also low GI. Adding these foods – as well as low GI carbohydrate foods – to meals will slow the absorption of the whole meal and reduce the GI of the entire meal.

How to exercise to beat cellulite

Tone up
The key is to include both strength (toning) training to build muscle as well as cardiovascular (aerobic) exercise to burn fat in your exercise programme. Strength training doesn't necessarily mean lifting heavy weights. It can be toning exercises (like press-ups and lunges) using your own body weight, light hand-held weights, exercise bands or tubes for resistance.

From fat to firm
Don't be afraid of adding strength exercises – you won't get muscle-bound or develop bigger legs! Just the opposite, in fact. As your muscles tone up, they'll become firmer and smaller. As you get older, collagen and elastin fibres become less elastic, which makes your fat more noticeable. But as you build muscle, the fibres are strengthened, reducing dimples, so the appearance of your cellulite will dramatically improve.

Up the burn
More muscle means more calories burned during activity as well as when resting. Every $^1/_2$ kg (1 lb) of muscle you add through exercise increases your metabolic rate by 30–40 calories a day. That's equal to 1200 extra calories a month, or a $^1/_2$-kg (1-lb) fat loss in three months without even changing your diet.

For the best fat-burning results, the American College of Sports Medicine recommends two strength training workouts a week in addition to three 20–40-minute cardiovascular (aerobic) workouts. Try swimming, power walking, running, cycling and group exercise classes. You'll find a detailed diet and exercise programme in the *30-Day Cellulite Plan* (Virgin Books).

CHAPTER 2
ALL IN A DAY'S EATING

Making small changes to the way you eat through the day can yield big results. You don't have to cut out all the foods you love – cut out only what doesn't benefit your body. There are literally hundreds of foods that you can include in your diet that will help you lose excess weight and combat cellulite. Here are 26 easy ways to achieve a leaner body. If you stick to them regularly, they'll help you get more of the cellulite superfoods you need into your diet.

Breakfast

NO BREAKFAST?
Don't even think about skipping breakfast. People who do are more likely to overeat later in the day and pile on unwanted pounds. Have a bowl of porridge or muesli with fruit (see pages 29–35), both are high in fibre.

FILL YOUR TANK
When you start your day off with a healthy, filling breakfast, you dramatically increase your chances of eating healthily throughout the day. You also fuel your body, so you feel happy and energised for the rest of the day. Studies show that when you eat a filling, high-fibre breakfast you'll eat 100–150 fewer calories for breakfast and lunch.

THINK FRUIT FIRST
Start with an orange, a grapefruit, some berries, or a sliced banana, then move on to the rest. At least you'll get a healthy dose of vitamins and fibre and it'll put you in a positive food mindset.

IN THE PINK
When you buy grapefruit, go for pink instead of white. It contains lycopene, the same phytonutrient that is found in tomatoes which can protect you from cancer and heart disease. Watermelon and guava also have some.

THE PITH OF THE MATTER
When peeling oranges and other citrus fruit, leave on some of the white pith under the rind. It's loaded with bioflavanoids, which fight off free radicals and also increase the absorption of vitamin C.

LIQUIDISE
No time to stop and eat? Grab a smoothie or whiz up your own with a blender or smoothie maker. Chop up a banana and blend with a handful of strawberries, a pot of low-fat yoghurt and a splash of skimmed milk.

DON'T TEMPT YOURSELF
If your normal route to work takes you past a bagel bar or a croissant shop, change your journey so that you bypass temptation.

Lunch

BRING IT IN
Bring your own lunch from home – you'll have more control over how many calories you eat. A study found that people who eat in restaurants daily consume 300 more calories a day than those who prepare their own food. Try hummus (ready-bought or Hummus with pine nuts, recipe page 37) with crudités and rye crackers or a healthy pasta salad (see Pasta and bean salad with grapes and black olives page 60).

START WITH SALAD
Eating a low-fat salad or a dish of fruit as a starter can cut the number of calories you eat in your main meal by 12 per cent, according to a study published in the *Journal of the American Dietetic Association*. All that fibre and water takes the edge off your appetite so you eat less of the higher calorie foods.

HAVE A SOUPER LUNCH

Starting your meal with a bowl of chunky soup can cut your calories by 20 per cent, according to a US study. The idea is that the fibre fills you up so you'll eat less of the higher calorie foods that follow.

EAT ALONE

One study found that people who dined in a group of two or more ate nearly twice as much on average as those who ate alone. But don't eat at your desk – when you eat as you're working or reading you don't notice what you're eating. Instead, go and sit somewhere else in the building, or even outside if the weather is reasonable.

MAKE YOUR SARNIE HEALTHIER

Can't say no to a deli sandwich? Make it healthier by opting for low GI rye bread, wholewheat pitta or multi-grain bread. They provide slow-releasing energy, which will make you feel satisfied longer and stop you feeling hungry. Fill with lots of chunky salad for added fibre and vitamins, and hummus, guacamole (avocado) or peanut butter for the heart-healthy unsaturated fats and vitamin E that they contain. Avoid white rolls, baguettes, bagels and ordinary sliced bread.

PLAN AHEAD

Plan your meals for the whole week. Sit down with a pen and paper and work out exactly what you need at the supermarket. Making a list before you go shopping means that you're more likely to stick to it, and planning ahead means you won't get home from work tired and hungry, only to discover there's nothing healthy in your fridge.

Dinner

JAZZ IT UP

Popping on a jazz or classical music CD can help you lose weight. Studies have found that listening to relaxing music while eating makes you chew more slowly and eat less than when listening to frantic tunes.

BE SIZE-WISE AT MEALTIMES

Stuff yourself with carbohydrate before bedtime and you definitely won't burn all the calories you've taken in. So, go easy on the pasta and potatoes and increase the vegetables, fresh fruit and lean protein. Replace half of your usual portion of pasta with veg and you won't eat any less food, just fewer calories. As a guide, a healthy serving of pasta or rice should be around 60 g (2 oz) (dry weight) and a serving of potato around 150 g (5 oz), or the size of two eggs.

VEG OUT

Aim for 3–5 portions of vegetables a day. They help you feel full without boosting your daily calorie intake. Three generous sprigs of broccoli contain just 45 calories, about the same as a nibble (one square) of chocolate.

SLOW DOWN

You'll eat 15 per cent fewer calories if you sit down and slow down your meal rather than eating on the hoof. Studies show that people eat up to 15 per cent more calories when they rush at mealtimes. Scoffing your meal means that your hypothalamus – the part of the brain that senses when you are full – doesn't receive the right signals and explains why you may feel hungrier sooner.

SWAP YOUR POTATO FOR A SWEET POTATO

Sweet potatoes have a much lower GI than ordinary potatoes, so they'll help you feel satisfied longer after your meal. What's more, one sweet potato gives you the recommended daily quota of heart-healthy omega-3 fatty acids. Studies show that diets rich in omega-3 fats also help speed weight loss, and boost your metabolism. You'll get the same benefits from a weekly portion of salmon, sardines or mackerel, 25 g (approximately one heaped tablespoon) of walnuts, or 1–2 omega-3-enriched eggs.

USE OIL SPRAY

Boiling, steaming, grilling and stir-frying are healthier ways to cook your food but you don't have to give up frying altogether. Using a one-cal spray instead of one teaspoon of oil saves about 50 calories.

EAT A LITTLE DESSERT

For many people a sweet dessert signals to your brain that the meal is over. Without it, you may not feel satisfied, which might leave you raiding the fridge later on for something to satisfy your sugar craving. Have some fresh fruit, a bowl of yoghurt topped with strawberries, blueberries, or sliced banana, or try one of the recipes in this book (see pages 120–133).

STEAL THE HIVE

Substituting honey for sugar in cooking saves calories as well adding antioxidants to protect your heart and health (see Baked apples with fruit and nuts, page 131). The American Chemical Society reports that honey contains substances which can help protect against cancer and ageing.

Snacks

GET FRUITY

Eating more fruit is one of the best things you can do for your health. Aim for 2–4 daily portions. Apart from the vital vitamins and minerals they provide, scientists know that fruit (and veg) contain a whole armoury of other substances that can protect you from heart disease and stroke, helping you lead a healthier and longer life.

EAT WHILE YOU WORK

Place at least two portions of fruit – apples, grapes, cherries, whatever fruit you like – on your desk. Promise to eat them before you leave work.

GO GREEN

Instead of coffee, go for a mug of green tea. It contains compounds called polyphenols that may increase calorie burn by as much as 4 per cent during the day.

QUICK FIX

Fancy something sweet? Replace sweets with collagen-strengthening fruits, such as berries, oranges, grapes, apricots, apples, plums, nectarines and cherries. Swap biscuits and cakes for lower GI, nutrient-packed nuts, seeds and dried fruits.

SAY NO TO LIQUID CALORIES

On average we consume 14 per cent of our daily calories in liquid form – sugary, fizzy drinks, alcohol, and coffee – so switching to water or herbal tea can save you more than 8000 calories – the equivalent of a weight loss of over 1 kg (2 lb) – a month.

DRINK WISELY

Not surprisingly, alcohol is the diet downfall of many people. A bottle of wine totals about 500 calories, so you can undo a whole day's good behaviour in just one boozy night. Alcohol can encourage fat storage. It's high in calories and puts undue stress on the liver. Alcohol calories can't be stored and have to be used as they are consumed – and this means that calories from other foods that are excess to requirements get stored as fat instead.

CHAPTER 3
CELLULITE SUPERFOODS

There's no such thing as a magical cellulite cure. No cream, pill, potion or gadget can melt away cellulite, but there are certain foods that are super-rich in nutrients which will help you win your battle against cellulite (fat). By including them in your daily diet, you will naturally be able to control your hunger and appetite, and so lose excess weight more easily. Importantly, they also provide a myriad of other health benefits, promote healthy skin and stronger collagen, thus helping improve the appearance of your cellulite.

Each superfood is really a category of foods, which have similar nutritional profiles so there are literally hundreds of fruit, vegetables, nuts, seeds, dairy products and other choices to satisfy your tastes. Incorporating these superfoods into your meals will help you beat cellulite from within. You'll find lots of inspiring recipes and ideas in the following chapters to help you add these superfoods to your diet.

The ten superfoods are:

1 **WALNUTS**
2 **BEANS**
3 **TOMATOES**
4 **BLUEBERRIES**
5 **MANGO**
6 **BROCCOLI**
7 **OATS**
8 **PUMPKIN SEEDS**
9 **ORANGES**
10 **LIVE BIO-YOGHURT**

1 Walnuts

Also: almonds, brazils, cashews, peanuts, pistachios, macadamia nuts, pine nuts and hazelnuts

Main nutrients

Omega-3 fatty acids	Fibre
Monounsaturated fatty acids	Potassium
Vitamin E	Vitamins B1, B2, B3, B6
Protein	Folate
Magnesium	

Key health benefits

Curb your hunger longer than other snacks
Regulate your appetite so you don't gain weight
Nurture your skin
Help combat wrinkles
Lower your cholesterol levels – especially the LDL ('bad') type
Reduce your risk of heart disease
Cut your chances of developing type-2 diabetes
Ward off cancer
Balance your mood
Help control blood pressure

HOW MUCH TO EAT?
One serving of 25 g (1 oz) at least five days a week

Walnuts have got a fattening image and most dieters give them a wide birth for fear of sabotaging their weight loss attempts. But that's completely wrong, according to the latest scientific research, which suggests that eating nuts can actually help you lose weight and keep it off (and that means less cellulite)!

People who include nuts as part of a balanced diet manage their weight more easily than those who don't, according to research carried out at Purdue University in the US. The reason is because nuts are filling and more satisfying to the appetite than most other foods. Researchers from the prestigious Harvard Medical School in the US found that eating nuts as part of a Mediterranean-style, moderate-fat diet helped people lose weight

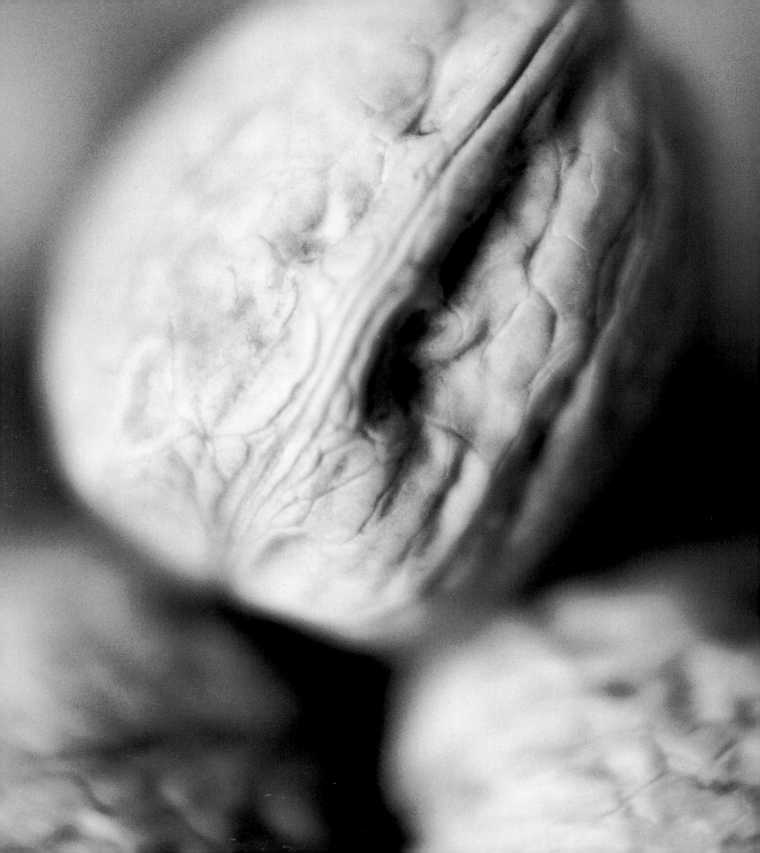

and keep it off longer than those who followed a traditional low-fat diet.

Nuts are good for your heart, too. A US study found that people who ate 30 g (1 oz) of nuts at least five times a week were up to 51 per cent less likely to develop heart disease. Amazingly, those who ate nuts just once a month still had some benefit.

The heart health benefits are partly explained by the high levels of 'good' monounsaturated fats and omega 3 fatty acids in nuts, as well as antioxidants called polyphenols. Omega-3s are found in especially high amounts in walnuts. They 'thin' the blood, preventing clots forming in blood vessels. They also have anti-inflammatory effects, preventing blood vessels from becoming inflamed and stopping blood flow; as well as lowering blood pressure.

Omega-3s also help strengthen your skin from within, improving its elasticity and reducing the formation of wrinkles. Smoother more elastic skin reduces the appearance of cellulite.

Eating nuts may even help you live longer. In a study of 11,000 people over 13 years at Oxford University, researchers found that eating nuts regularly significantly reduced the risk of death from any cause.

Including nuts in your daily diet reduces LDL ('bad' cholesterol) by 35 per cent, according to a study at the University of Toronto, in Canada, and lowers the risk of type-2 diabetes by 21 per cent according to a study at Harvard University.

All nuts are a rich source of fibre, vitamin E (which helps keep the heart healthy), B vitamins (which help release energy from food), folate (also lowers the risk of heart disease and helps prevent cancer) and magnesium (important for healthy bones and nerve and muscle function). Almonds provide high amounts of calcium. The ubiquitous peanut is an excellent source of the antioxidant resveratrol (which is also found in red wine), which further boosts your defences against cancer and heart disease.

Tip: Nuts turn rancid quite quickly, so buy them from a shop with a fast turnover. Avoid nuts that have a bitter or sharp smell as this indicates rancidity. Keep nuts in an airtight container in a cool place. You can roast them to bring out their full flavour. Spread the nuts on a baking tray and place in a 170–180°C/325–250°F/Gas mark 3–4 oven for 5–10 minutes (depending on the type of nut) until they are lightly golden.

2 Beans
Red kidney beans, aduki beans, chickpeas, haricot beans, cannelloni beans, borlotti beans, red, green and brown lentils

Main nutrients
Protein	Iron
Complex carbohydrates	Potassium
Fibre	Magnesium
B vitamins	Folate

Key health benefits
Help you manage your weight
Regulate your appetite
Lower your cholesterol levels – especially the LDL ('bad') type
Cut your risk of heart disease
Helps control type-2 diabetes
Prevent cancer
Balance your mood
Helps control blood pressure

HOW MUCH TO EAT?
One to four servings a week

Beans fill you up – as anyone who's ever eaten them knows! This is what makes them so good for weight (cellulite) loss. They provide lots of bulk without a lot of calories. When you include beans and lentils in your diet, you tend to get full before you get fat. The high-fibre content of beans and their low GI help to control blood sugar and stave off hunger, while still giving you longer lasting energy. The fibre in beans also helps to keep 'bad' LDL cholesterol levels down while boosting 'good' HDL cholesterol.

Beans are a great low-fat source of protein. They are rich in the amino acid lysine, which is lacking in most other plant proteins (such as cereals). Combining them with pasta, oats or rice therefore balances the amino acids of the meal so you end up with a higher quality protein.

Beans can also help cut your heart disease risk. A study of nearly 10,000 men and women found that those who ate beans or lentils at least four times a week had a 22 per cent lower risk of heart disease compared to those who ate them less than once a week. They also had lower blood pressure, lower blood cholesterol levels and a lower chance of having diabetes.

Beans are particularly good for diabetics who need to control their blood sugar levels through diet. They provide steady slow-burning energy due to their high content of soluble fibre.

There is also good evidence that beans can help prevent cancer. This is thought to be due to their high content of phytates, compounds that combat certain cancers, and phytoestrogens (lignins), which have been shown to reduce the risk of cancers that are related to oestrogen levels, particularly breast cancer.

Beans and lentils are rich in iron which is essential for transporting oxygen around the body, as well as B vitamins, zinc and magnesium.

Tip: Ideally, use dried beans and lentils soaked and then cooked according to the packet instructions. But, for convenience, tinned versions are almost as good. Choose beans canned without added salt and sugar, otherwise rinse them in a sieve under running water for 20–30 seconds. This eliminates around 40 per cent of the salt. If you're not used to eating beans, incorporate them gradually in to your diet in small amounts so that your body becomes accustomed to them and experiences less wind and discomfort.

3 Tomatoes

Main nutrients
Lycopene	Lutein
Alpha- and beta-carotene	Potassium
Vitamin C	Fibre

Key health benefits
Prevent certain cancers
Reduce heart disease risk
Protect your skin from ultra violet light
Help combat wrinkles

HOW MUCH TO EAT?
Three to four servings a week

Tomatoes are used in a lot of traditional Mediterranean dishes and sauces. This helps to explain why people who eat a Mediterranean diet have the lowest chances of heart disease and cancer in Europe. The more you can incorporate them into your diet the better.

So, what's the big news with tomatoes? For starters, they are stuffed with phytonutrients (plant nutrients), the most potent being lycopene. This natural pigment is responsible for the red colour in tomatoes. Research shows that people who regularly eat tomatoes and tomato products have a lower risk of certain cancers, particularly prostate cancer and that a high lycopene level in the body is associated with a lower risk of heart disease.

A study at the University of Toronto found that women who regularly consume tomatoes and tomato products are less likely to develop breast cancer. A study of European men showed that those with high levels of lycopene in their bodies had half the heart attack risk as men with low levels. It's also been linked to a reduced risk of cancer of the stomach, colon and rectum.

Normally, nutritionists advise eating fresh fruit and vegetables. But lycopene is more easily absorbed into the body when the tomato has been cooked or processed, which means that tinned tomatoes, passata (sieved tomatoes), tomato pasta sauce and tomato soup are a better source than raw tomatoes.

Amazingly, lycopene can also act as an internal sun block. Working together with the other antioxidant nutrients in tomatoes, it can help protect your skin from the damaging effects of ultra-violet light. However, you should still wear sunscreen at all times in the sun.

Apart from lycopene, tomatoes also contain high levels of alpha- and beta-carotene and vitamin C. These vitamins help boost the immune system as well as combating the free radicals that are linked with heart disease and cancer.

But it's the combination of the nutrients in tomatoes that appear to have such a powerful anti-cancer effect. A study carried out at the Harvard Medical School in the US showed that eating two servings of cooked tomatoes per week significantly reduced cancer risk.

Tip: Choose the reddest tomatoes you can find. Vine-ripened tomatoes contain more vitamin C than most ordinary tomatoes, which are picked under-ripe. Serve tomatoes with a drizzle of olive oil to enhance lycopene absorption. If fresh ones aren't available, use tinned ones. Even tomato soup and pasta sauce are full of the goodness of tomatoes.

4 Blueberries
Also: Strawberries, raspberries, blackberries, and cranberries

Main nutrients

Antioxidant phytonutrients	Fibre
Anthocyanin and ellagic acid	Folate
Vitamin C	Potassium
Vitamin E	

Key health benefits
Improve condition of the skin
Strengthen collagen
Reduce wrinkles
Lower the risk of heart disease and stroke
Help combat cancer
Anti-aging
Protect against degenerative eye disease and cataracts

HOW MUCH TO EAT?
Three to four servings (85 g/3 oz) a week

They're delicious, energising and good for you. Berries, and blueberries in particular, are true superfoods, ranking above all other fruits for their remarkable health benefits.

Berries are densely packed with vitamins, antioxidants and other phytonutrients (health-promoting plant nutrients). Researchers in the US compared the antioxidant power of all fruits and vegetables and ranked cranberries and blueberries at the top of the league table for antioxidant power, closely followed by blackberries, raspberries and strawberries.

The main antioxidant in these super-berries is a class of compounds called anthocyanins – it's the pigment that makes blueberries blue, blackberries purple and raspberries red. But, what's important is that anthocyanins neutralise free-radical damage to cells and tissues and help stop cancer and heart disease in their tracks. Blueberries, raspberries and blackberries also contain ellagic acid (mainly in their seeds), another powerful antioxidant that fights cancer. Blueberries also contain high levels of resveratrol, which as mentioned before is also found in red wine and grapes – another powerful antioxidant that helps combat free radicals

So how does all this help combat cellulite? Well, eating berries regularly will improve the condition of your skin and therefore reduce the bumpy appearance of your cellulite. This incredible ability is due to the both the anthocyanins and the vitamin C contained in the berries. These two work together to strengthen blood capillaries and improve blood flow to those fatty areas. This means more oxygen flows around those areas and there is better removal of waste products. Anthocyanins and vitamin C also boost your body's production of collagen, an important building block of the connective tissue separating your fat cells. Weak and damaged connective tissue between fat cells is responsible for the dimples and irregularities characteristic of cellulite.

Here are some more good reasons to tuck into berries:
They help reduce the risk of degenerative eye diseases and cataracts. One study at the USDA Human Nutrition Centre on Aging at Tufts University found that eating blueberries can help slow down the aging process. University of California scientists have discovered that the antioxidants in blueberries reduce the build-up of 'bad' LDL cholesterol. A report in 2004 by researchers for the Department of Agriculture in the United States showed that the compound pterostilbene, which is found in blueberries, could be as effective as commercial drugs in lowering cholesterol. The same compound, similar to that found in red wine, has already been shown to help prevent type 2 diabetes and some cancers.

Finally, blueberries and cranberries have unique 'anti-stick' properties that help ward off urinary tract infections, ulcers and gum disease. Fresh cranberries, unfortunately, are very sour, but you can get all the heart-protective and 'anti-stick' benefits by drinking cranberry juice.

Tip: If you can't always buy fresh, try dried berries. Blueberries, cranberries and cherries are perfect for snacking or adding to low-fat muffins, home-made bread and pancakes. They retain all the health benefits of fresh berries – the antioxidant phytonutrients and anthocyanins are actually concentrated – although the vitamin C content is lower.

5 Mango
Also: Papaya

Main nutrients
Beta-carotene and other carotenoids	Fibre
	Vitamin E
Vitamin C	Potassium

Key health benefits
Improves skin appearance
Helps protect against ultra violet light
Strengthens blood vessels
Improves appetite control
Reduces heart disease risk
Helps combat certain cancers

HOW MUCH TO EAT?
One to two servings (half a mango) a week

It's not just the wonderful aromatic taste that makes mangos so special, they're also crammed full of nutrients. They are the best fruit source of the antioxidant carotenoids, such as beta-carotene, as well as a useful source of vitamin C, vitamin E and potassium.

Here's how eating more mangos will benefit your cellulite:
Beta-carotene in mangos promotes healthy new cells and boosts the natural elasticity of the skin, creating smoother and more evenly textured skin even in cellulite-affected areas. The vitamin C in mangos is good for making healthy blood vessels and strengthening collagen, the cement between the fat cells.

Mangos could also help reduce your chances of damaging your skin when it is exposed to the sun. The US National Cancer Institute recommends 6000 micrograms of beta-carotene daily – mangos have 683 micrograms per 100 g (3 oz).

Mangos are one of the few fruit sources of vitamin E, an important antioxidant that helps to fight damaging free radicals in the body as well as boosting the action of disease-fighting antibodies.

The high levels of soluble fibre in mangos help keep blood cholesterol levels low and your heart healthy, too. Fibre also helps balance blood sugar levels and stave off hunger pangs – helping you control your appetite easily and manage your weight.

Both mango and papaya contain the phytonutrient beta-cryptoxanthin which is a powerful antioxidant that helps prevent cancer. A 15-year study of 15,000 women found that those who consumed high levels of cryptoxanthin-rich food had a lower risk of cervical cancer. Researchers in New Zealand also found that people who ate mangos and papayas regularly were less likely to develop cancer of the colon.

> Tip: The easiest way to eat a mango is to slice it lengthwise as close to the stone as possible, on each side of the stone. Score the flesh into cubes, without cutting the skin and then turn inside out and cut the flesh off.

6 Broccoli
Also: Brussels sprouts, cabbage, spinach , curly kale, cauliflower, bok choi (pak choi)

Main nutrients

Sulphoraphane	Beta-carotene
Indoles	Fibre
Vitamin C	Calcium

Key health benefits
Helps weight loss
Fights cancer
Helps prevent heart disease and stroke
Helps strengthen bones

HOW MUCH TO EAT?
One serving (85 g/3 oz) five to seven times a week

Most people have bad memories of being forced to 'eat their greens', but now it turns out that your mother was right all along – green vegetables really are very good for us. And the king of them all turns out to be broccoli. This superfood is full of nutrients that help to prevent cancer, heart disease and osteoporosis – and even aid weight loss.

Broccoli and other members of the cruciferous family are rich in the soluble type of fibre, which helps slow down the absorption of carbohydrates from the intestines and promote stable blood sugar levels. And this means less hunger, better appetite control and easier weight loss. All good news where cellulite is concerned.

But broccoli has a myriad of other health benefits. Along with the other members of its family, broccoli is one of the most powerful weapons in the fight against cancer. A study of over 47,000 men at Harvard Medical School in the US was the first to establish a link between eating broccoli and reducing your risk of the disease. Since then, nearly 100 studies have confirmed these findings. Just one daily serving (two broccoli florets) gives you significant protection from cancers of the lungs, breast, stomach, colon and rectum. How come? It's all down to two incredible sulphur-containing compounds in these vegetables – sulforaphane and indoles. Sulphoraphane boosts the body's enzymes that kill abnormal cells as well as actually killing pre-cancerous cells.

And the fight doesn't stop there. There's also loads of vitamin C and beta-carotene in cruciferous veggies, two powerful antioxidant nutrients that stop the damage caused by free radicals. It's this damage that leads to cancer. One serving (85 g) of cooked broccoli provides approximately 100 per cent of the recommended daily requirement for vitamin C.

Broccoli also helps protect against heart disease and stroke. This is due to the combined effect of all those antioxidant compounds packed in this humble vegetable – flavanoids, carotenoids, folate, fibre, vitamin C and potassium. They all interact to prevent damage to the artery walls that ultimately lead to heart disease.

Folate, a B vitamin, has a further benefit. It lowers homocysteine (a by-product of protein metabolism) levels in the blood; high levels are associated with heart disease. It is also important for preventing neural tube defects such as spinal bifida in newborn babies.

Then there's the calcium, albeit in smallish quantities, but the accompanying vitamins and minerals mean that the calcium is absorbed well. Calcium helps build strong bones.

For an added health boost, try broccoli sprouts (sprouted broccoli seeds, which look like alfalfa sprouts), which you can grow in jars or trays from broccoli seeds (from health food stores). They contain up to 50 times more sulphoraphane than mature broccoli. Add them to salads or sandwiches.

As for the rest of the cruciferous family, spinach is excellent for preserving your eyesight. It contains lutein and zeaxanthin, two powerful antioxidants that help prevent age-related eye diseases.

Ever wondered why Brussels sprouts have got that slightly bitter taste and pungent smell? Well, its due to a compound called sinigrin (an isothiocyanate) which fights cancer by triggering the death of pre-cancerous cells. Even one serving (nine) of sprouts can have this effect!

If you've never tried bok choi (pak choi) – also known as Chinese cabbage – here's a good reason to buy it: one serving will give you a quarter of your daily vitamin A needs and one third of your vitamin C, along with cancer-busting flavanoids, isothiocyanates and dithiolthione.

Tip: When buying broccoli, look for young broccoli (which doesn't have a strong odour) and choose tight, deeply coloured and dense florets. The deeper the colour the more phytonutrients. Yellowing florets are signs that the broccoli is old and has lost a lot of its nutrients. When cooking broccoli, don't discard the stalk – it is rich in nutrients – just slice it up and steam it along with the florets.

7 Oats
Also: All wholegrains – brown rice, rye, barley, wheat, buckwheat, quinoa, millet

Main nutrients

Insoluble and soluble fibre	Iron
Complex carbohydrates	Zinc
Phytic acid	Vitamin E
Antioxidant phytonutrients	Selenium

Key health benefits
Stabilise blood sugar levels
Reduce hunger
Help manage type 2 diabetes
Lower cholesterol
Reduce colon cancer risk
Lower risk of heart disease and stroke

HOW MUCH TO EAT?
At least three servings of whole grains a day

It's a myth that whole grains are fattening. This stems from the fact that most people eat refined rather than whole grains, that is white bread and pasta, cakes, biscuits and buns, which are low in fibre and often loaded with sugars and fat. Whole grains, on the other hand, are highly satisfying as well as very nutritious. Because of their naturally high fibre content, you'll get full before you get fat! A 2000 study published in the *Journal of Nutrition* concluded that high-fibre foods such as whole grains help people lose weight and keep it off in the long term.

Whole grains provide both insoluble and soluble fibre. Each type will benefit your health. Insoluble fibre promotes a healthy digestive system and has been linked with a lower risk of bowel cancer. A study published in the scientific journal *Food Chemistry* in 2004 found that wheat bran's antioxidant power is 20 times higher than refined wheat flour.

Soluble fibre helps lower blood cholesterol levels and reduces the risk of heart disease. A US study published in the medical journal *Circulation* concluded that adding 3 g of soluble oat fibre to your daily diet lowers 'bad' LDL cholesterol by 10 per cent. This is due mainly to beta-glucan, a type of soluble fibre, which attracts cholesterol-based bile acids in the intestine and carries them out of the body. Cholesterol is then taken from the blood to make more bile acids and so cholesterol levels are lowered.

An international research review published in 2005 found that people who eat wholegrain foods regularly have a 20–40 per cent lower risk of heart disease and stroke compared with those who rarely eat wholegrain foods. The Australian researchers concluded that eating four servings of wholegrains is comparable to the effect you get from the powerful 'statin' drugs that doctors prescribe to lower blood cholesterol levels.

A US study in 2004 involving 330,000 adults concluded that for every 10 g of cereal fibre consumed a day (equivalent to three slices of wholegrain bread) the risk of death from heart disease was cut by 25 per cent. They also found a 27 per cent decrease in the risk of dying from heart disease. Plus the new 2005 US dietary guidelines recommend everyone should eat a minimum three servings (equivalent to three slices of wholemeal bread) a day.

Oats are particularly useful for managing type 2 diabetes as they stabilise blood sugar, but including them in your diet regularly will reduce the chances of developing it in the first place, according to a 2003 study published in the *American Journal of Clinical Nutrition*.

Oats and other whole grains also help lower the risk of colon cancer. They contain phytic acid which decreases the rate at which cancer cells spread and enhances the immune system.

As well as the fibre benefits of wholegrains, scientists are also studying the role of phytonutrients in whole grains and how they help prevent disease. Wheat contains lutein, zeaxanthin and beta-cryptoxanthin, potent antioxidants that protect against cancer.

Whole grains also supply iron (which transports oxygen to your muscle cells), zinc (for making new cells, healing and fighting infection), vitamin E (strengthens the immune system) and selenium (which helps mop up free radicals). But it's the synergy of nutrients in whole grains that make them an outstanding superfood.

> Tip: For a quick breakfast, instant oats provide all the nutritional benefits of whole oats. The oats are pre-cooked and pulverised to a finer 'flour', which increases slightly their glycaemic index. But they're still healthier than refined cereals. Choose the unsweetened, unflavoured variety and add fresh or dried fruit for flavour.

8 Pumpkin seeds

Also: Flaxseeds (linseeds), sesame seeds, pumpkin seed oil, flaxseed oil, sesame oil

Main nutrients

Omega-3 fatty acids	Magnesium
Monounsaturated fatty acids	Iron
Vitamin E	Fibre
Protein	Selenium

Key health benefits

Curb your hunger
Regulate your appetite
Healthy skin
Lower your cholesterol levels – especially the LDL ('bad') type
Reduce your risk of heart disease
Reduce cancer risk

HOW MUCH TO EAT?

One tablespoon of seeds or their oils (15 g / ¹/₂ oz) a day

Ditch the biscuits and crisps and, instead, tuck in to a small handful of pumpkin seeds.

Contrary to the myth, seeds won't make you gain weight. Quite the reverse, in fact, as they are so satisfying, helping to curb your hunger more effectively than sugary snacks. They are high in protein and healthy fats, which means they have one of the lowest glycaemic index values of all foods, promoting steady blood sugar levels and low insulin levels. This results in sustained energy with minimal fat storage.

The seeds and oils in this category are rich sources of omega-3 fatty acids, namely alpha-linolenic acid (ALA). Research suggests that omega-3 fatty acids may help regulate your body's blood sugar levels by increasing insulin sensitivity and boosting your metabolic rate, both of which will help prevent weight gain.

Most people eat ten times more omega-6 fatty acids (found in processed foods containing cooking oils and margarine) than omega-3 fatty acids, while a 3:1 ratio would be a healthier balance.

The omega-3 fatty acids that are present in your brain's cell walls aid the action of mood-enhancing chemicals such as serotonin, which directly improves the way you feel. Omega-3s have anti-inflammatory and anti-clotting properties. If they're outweighed by omega-6s, you may be more prone to heart disease, asthma, eczema and cancer. To shift the balance, tuck into more pumpkin and flax seeds (and their oils).

A higher omega-3 consumption may also help reduce pain in people with rheumatoid arthritis and reduce the inflammation of airway cells that trigger asthma attacks.

Omega-3s are also needed to keep all the cells in your skin watertight, so if you don't get enough in your diet, you risk dry, flaky, lifeless skin.

Like nuts, seeds are also rich in heart-healthy monounsaturated fats, which reduce 'bad' LDL cholesterol and cut heart disease and stroke risk.

Seeds and their oils owe much of their heart health benefits to their high levels of phytosterols, plant chemicals that can help reduce cholesterol levels. Phytosterols have a similar structure to cholesterol and they compete for absorption in the intestine, As a result, less cholesterol is absorbed and cholesterol levels in the bloodstream are lowered.

Linseeds contain lignins, which protect against free radical damage and are also believed to prevent cancer of the breast and colon. Linseeds also help to keep the bowel healthy. They may also help manage menopausal symptoms.

And just to complete the nutritional picture, seeds and their oils are also packed with vitamin E, protein, iron, folate, potassium, zinc, selenium, magnesium and fibre. Note that pumpkin seeds and oil are richer in iron than other varieties

Tip: Choose pre-cracked linseeds or grind them yourself. This breaks down the tough outer husk, releasing the beneficial oils and nutrients so they can be absorbed by the body.

9 Oranges

Also: Satsumas, clementines, mandarins, kiwi fruit, grapefruit, lemons, limes

Main nutrients

Vitamin C	Folic acid
Bioflavanoids	Fibre
Hesperitin	potassium

Key health benefits

Strengthen collagen
Improve circulation
Strengthen blood vessels
Lower risk of certain cancers
Reduce heart disease risk

HOW MUCH TO EAT?
One citrus fruit a day

Santa Claus was doing you a big favour when he left a small orange at the bottom of your stocking as a child. That symbolic fruit is a powerhouse of vitamins and phytonutrients that boosts your immunity, protects your health and – now as an adult – may even reduce your cellulite.

Oranges and other citrus fruit are rich in vitamin C, which, among other things, helps to boost the body's production of collagen. This, in turn, helps reduce cellulite because strong collagen supports the fat cells, stopping them becoming misshapen. Weak collagen is one of the causes of the dimply fat. Strong collagen is also important for healthy skin and defending the body against bacteria.

Vitamin C together with the bioflavanoids present in citrus fruit, also strengthens blood capillaries. This improves circulation generally in the body but especially in fatty tissue, which is prone to sluggish circulation. Boosting blood flow improves oxygen and nutrient delivery to the cells and ensures the efficient removal of toxins and waste products.

Bioflavanoids are powerful antioxidants that help protect the body from free radical damage. They are concentrated in the pith and membranes of oranges so it's better to eat the whole fruit than to drink the juice. They work with other phytonutrients in oranges to maximise the absorption and benefits of vitamin C. Citrus fruit protect the body through their antioxidant properties by strengthening the immune system, inhibiting tumour growth and preventing pre-cancerous cells turning cancerous.

Unbelievably, there are more than 60 different bioflavanoids in oranges – all with impressive anti-cancer and blood clot inhibiting properties. But the most important is hesperidin. In tests, hesperidin has been found to inhibit breast cancer cell growth. An Australian study, based on 48 international studies, found that people who eat citrus fruit regularly have up to 50 per cent less risk of developing stomach cancer. Bioflavanoids also have a remarkable ability to absorb ultra-violet light, protect DNA and stop cancer-causing agents. A study on mice found that citrus bioflavanoids helped to reduce the development of skin cancer.

One extra serving of citrus fruit a day – on top of the recommended five a day – could also reduce the risk of stroke by 19 per cent. It's the combined effects of the bioflavanoids, vitamin C and the fibre in these fruit that make them such powerful superfoods. Pectin, the main type of fibre in citrus fruit, helps lower cholesterol and is helpful in stabilising blood sugar.

Oranges also help protect your heart because of their high folate levels which lower the concentration of homocysteine – an amino acid by-product of protein metabolism that is implicated in heart disease – in the blood. Studies have shown that people who consume the most folate have the lowest risk of heart attack and stroke.

Tip: Make use of the rind of citrus fruit too. It contains limonene, an antioxidant that can stop cancer in its earliest stages. Add thinly pared zest to salad dressings, low fat muffins or drinks. Buy organic and unwaxed fruit if possible, otherwise wash it thoroughly to remove pesticide residues, wax and dirt.

10 Live bio-yoghurt

Main nutrients

Calcium	Vitamin B12
Protein	Pro-biotic bacteria cultures
Riboflavin	

Key health benefits

Aids weight loss
Helps reduce cellulite
Promotes a healthy digestive system
Reduces transit time
Maintains the immune system
Combats fungal infections
Prevents constipation

HOW MUCH TO EAT?
One to two servings (125 g/4 oz) a day

Yoghurt has long been hailed as a health food but new research on probiotics and gut health, and its potential role in weight loss elevates it to the ranks of a superfood.

What's fast emerging from the research is yoghurt's ability to help you lose weight – and that includes cellulite, of course. A study carried out at the University of Tennessee in 2004 found that people who included dairy foods in their diet for 24 weeks lost up to 4.5 kg (10 lb) more weight than those who ate a normal diet, containing the same number of calories. What's more, the dairy eaters lost 66 per cent of fat from their belly, compared with only 8 per cent in those on the normal diet. Another study by the North American Association for the Study of Obesity concluded that women who ate at least three servings of low-fat dairy products a day were 80 per cent less likely to become obese than those who ate fewer dairy products.

Experts suggest that it's the high calcium content in dairy foods that speeds up the body's metabolism, causing it to burn more calories and so help you shed weight. If you don't get enough calcium from food, the body begins conserving calcium, prompting it to produce higher levels of a hormone called calcitriol, which then triggers a higher level of fat in fat cells.

The best yoghurt choice, though, is live bio-yoghurt (or probiotic) yoghurt because it also helps promote a healthy gut.

Live bio-yoghurt contains health-boosting lactobacillus and bifida bacteria which, if consumed regularly enough, can change the balance of bacteria in your bowel or colon. A healthy digestive system should be teaming with these 'friendly' probiotic bacteria – they aid efficient digestion and the absorption of food, inhibit the growth of harmful bacteria (such as salmonella and E coli, which can cause food poisoning) and help to combat the negative effects of stress, alcohol, highly processed foods and the imbalance that can be caused in the body by drugs such as antibiotics. As if all that isn't impressive enough, they also help to maintain the immune system, combat fungal infections, such as thrush, and they can reduce the need for antibiotics to fight infections. Probiotics replace beneficial bacteria needed by the body that can be killed off by antibiotic treatment.

If you suffer from a sluggish gut or are prone to constipation, eating live bio-yoghurt regularly will alleviate your symptoms and also prevent related conditions like haemorrhoids and diverticular disease. Bifidus bacteria can speed up the time it takes for food to pass through the digestive system – basically, optimising your transit time. This means food can be properly digested and absorbed, with minimal bloating and discomfort caused by excessive gas.

People who are intolerant to milk and other dairy products often find yoghurt acceptable.

Tip: Despite its healthy image, not all yoghurt is healthy. Most varieties are laden with added sugar and artificial additives. So choose plain or 'natural' varieties from the chill cabinet (this means that its 'live') and then check the label for the words 'bio', 'live' and ideally bifidus bacteria. Check that it contains no added sugar and no artificial colours or sweeteners. Add chopped fresh fruit or dried fruit to plain yoghurt or stir in a tablespoon of chopped nuts or seeds for an added nutrient boost.

CHAPTER 4
BREAKFASTS

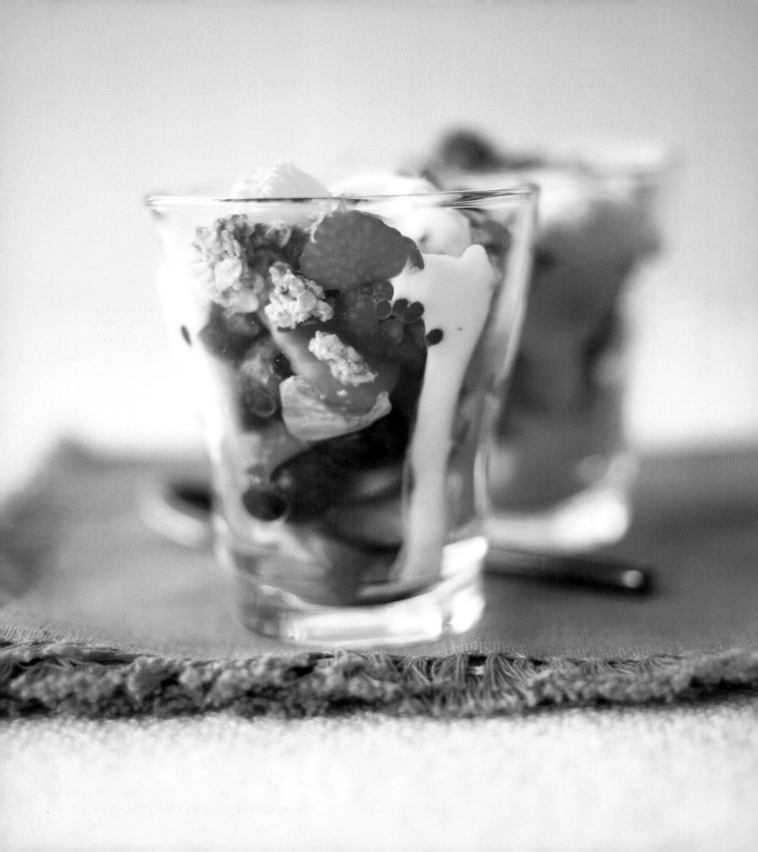

BREAKFAST CRUMBLE

MAKE 2 SERVINGS

I think this breakfast is more like a pudding so it's hard to believe that it's so good for you. It's a delicious way of getting one or two portions of your five-a-day target for fruit and vegetables.

1 peach
1 orange
125 g (4 oz) berries, e.g. strawberries, blueberries, raspberries
A little fruit juice
85 g (3 oz) crunchy cereal (granola)
2–3 tablespoons (30–45 ml) live bio-yoghurt

▸ Slice the peach and divide the orange into segments. Mix with the berries then divide the fruit into two bowls. Pour over a little fruit juice, just enough to moisten the fruit. Top each bowl with half the crunchy cereal and serve with a dollop of yoghurt.

HEALTH STATISTICS
Berries are brim-full of vitamin C, anthocyanins (powerful antioxidants) and cancer-protective ellagic acid. The crunchy cereal contains oats, which are good sources of soluble fibre and provide slow-releasing energy. The bio-yoghurt provides calcium protein and friendly bacteria that help promote a healthy gut.

NUTRITIONAL ANALYSIS (PER SERVING):

Calories 241 kcal	Carbohydrate 47 g
Protein 8.5 g	Total sugars* 30 g
Fat 3.3 g	Fibre 2.9 g
Saturates 0.7 g	Salt 0.2 g

* total sugars includes sugars found naturally in foods

PORRIDGE WITH FRUIT

MAKES 2 SERVINGS

Starting the day with a bowl of porridge gives me a fantastic energy boost. I like to add chopped fresh fruit – try sliced banana, blueberries, strawberries, clementine segments or any other fruit that takes your fancy.

85 g (3 oz) rolled porridge oats
125 ml (4 fl oz) skimmed soya, rice, sesame or almond milk
125 ml (4 fl oz) water
2 tablespoons (30 ml) raisins, sultanas, dried apricots or dates
125 g (4 oz) fresh fruit (see above)
1 tablespoon (15 ml) honey

▸ Mix the oats, milk and water in a saucepan. Bring to the boil and simmer for 4–5 minutes, stirring frequently.
▸ Stir in the dried fruit. Spoon into bowls, drizzle over the honey and top with fresh fruit.

HEALTH STATISTICS
Oats are rich in soluble fibre, which is excellent for improving digestion and lowering blood cholesterol, as well as iron, B vitamins, vitamin E and zinc. They provide slow-released energy to sustain you through the morning. The dried and fresh fruit provide extra fibre and vitamins.

NUTRITIONAL ANALYSIS (PER SERVING):

Calories 261 kcal	Carbohydrate 51 g
Protein 7.7 g	Total sugars* 24 g
Fat 4.2 g	Fibre 4.0 g
Saturates 0.8 g	Salt 0.1 g

* total sugars includes sugars found naturally in foods

LOW-FAT BLUEBERRY MUFFINS WITH APPLE SPREAD

MAKES 12 MUFFINS

When you haven't got time to sit down for breakfast, these fruity antioxidant-packed muffins make the perfect breakfast on the move. Keep a supply in the freezer, defrost a couple overnight then simply grab and go in the morning.

225g (8 oz) wholemeal self-raising flour
40g (1½oz) clear honey
1 tablespoon (15 ml) sunflower oil
1 egg
200ml (7 fl oz) skimmed or non-dairy milk
125g (4oz) fresh or frozen blueberries

FOR THE APPLE SPREAD:
2 large cooking apples
60 g (2 oz) raisins
1 tablespoon (15 ml) clear honey
Pinch of ground cinnamon
25 g (1 oz) olive oil spread

▸ Preheat the oven to 200°C/400°F/Gas mark 6.
▸ Put the flour in a bowl, then add the honey, oil, egg and milk. Mix well, then stir in the blueberries.
▸ Fill a 12-compartment deep muffin tray with 12 paper cases. Spoon the mixture into the paper cases.
▸ Bake for approximately 15 minutes until golden brown.

TO MAKE THE APPLE SPREAD:
▸ Peel, core and slice the apples then place in a saucepan with a little water. Add the raisins, honey and cinnamon and cook the apple mixture over a gentle heat until mushy. Remove from the heat, beat the mixture to a pulp then stir in the olive oil spread. Chill in the fridge, where it will thicken a little.
▸ Serve the muffins warm with the spread.

HEALTH STATISTICS
Substituting wholemeal flour for the usual white flour adds extra fibre as well as B vitamins and iron. The muffins contain significantly lower levels of fat and sugar compared to ordinary muffins and the apple spread provides vitamin C, potassium and the cancer-beating antioxidant, quercetin.

NUTRITIONAL ANALYSIS (PER MUFFIN):

Calories 91 kcal	Carbohydrate 16 g
Protein 3.7 g	Total sugars* 4.2 g
Fat 1.9 g	Fibre 2.0 g
Saturates 0.3 g	Salt 0.1 g

* total sugars includes sugars found naturally in foods

FOR THE APPLE SPREAD:
Nutritional Analysis (per serving):

Calories 38 kcal	Carbohydrate 6.8 g
Protein 0.2 g	Total sugars* 6.8 g
Fat 1.3 g	Fibre 0.5 g
Saturates 0.2 g	Salt 0.1 g

* total sugars includes sugars found naturally in foods

GRANOLA WITH APPLE AND APRICOT COMPOTE

MAKES 2 SERVINGS

This homemade granola is highly nutritious and contains much less sugar and oil than shop-bought versions. You can make larger quantities and store in an airtight container for up to four weeks.

FOR THE GRANOLA:
2 teaspoons (10 ml) clear honey
2 teaspoons (10 ml) sunflower oil
2 teaspoons (10 ml) lemon juice
½ teaspoon (2.5 ml) ground cinnamon
60 g (2 oz) oats
15 g (½ oz) sesame seeds
25g (1 oz) hazelnuts, crushed
25 g (1 oz) mixed dried berries (or raisins)

FOR THE APPLE AND APRICOT COMPOTE:
60 g (2oz) ready-to-eat dried apricots
1 apple, peeled, cored and chopped
1 teaspoon (5 ml) clear honey
Juice of ½ lemon
½ teaspoon (2.5 ml) ground cinnamon

▸ Heat the oven to 150°C/275°F/Gas Mark 1.
▸ Combine the honey, oil, lemon juice, vanilla and cinnamon in a saucepan, then warm over a gentle heat until evenly mixed. Turn off the heat then mix in the oats, sesame seeds and hazelnuts.
▸ Spread out the mixture on a non-stick baking tray and bake in the oven for 50–60 minutes, stirring occasionally until golden brown.
▸ Cool and then mix in the dried berries. Store in an airtight container until ready to serve.

FOR THE COMPOTE:
▸ Put the apricots, apples, honey, lemon juice and cinnamon in a saucepan together with approximately 4 tablespoons of water. Stir and bring to the boil. Reduce the heat and simmer for 10 minutes until the fruit is tender. Allow to cool.
▸ To serve: spoon a dollop of plain bio-yoghurt into a bowl and top with the apple and apricot compote and a generous sprinkling of granola.

HEALTH STATISTICS
Oats are rich in soluble fibre and provide slow-released energy as well as plenty of B vitamins and iron. Hazelnuts and sesame seeds provide protein, calcium, zinc and healthy monounsaturated oils. The apple and apricot compote provide extra fibre, beta-carotene and iron.

NUTRITIONAL ANALYSIS:

Calories 429 kcal	Carbohydrate 55 g
Protein 8.5 g	Total sugars* 33 g
Fat 21 g	Fibre 6.5 g
Saturates 1.9 g	Salt 0.1 g

* total sugars includes sugars found naturally in foods

OAT MUESLI WITH BERRIES

MAKES 2 SERVINGS

This muesli is very easy to make. I like to soak the oats overnight – they're nicer when they're soft and have absorbed the flavours of the dried fruit. Alternatively, you can use a ready-made muesli base then add your own nuts and fruit. I think blueberries – when you can get them – make a delicious, indulgent topping.

85 g (3 oz) porridge oats
150 ml (¼ pint) skimmed soya, rice, almond or oat 'milk'
2 tablespoons (30 ml) raisins (or other dried fruit)
2 tablespoons (30 ml) chopped brazils or walnuts
1 tablespoon (15 ml) ground linseeds (optional)
125 g (4oz) blueberries, raspberries or strawberries

▸ In a large bowl, mix together the oats (or other flakes), milk, dried fruit, nuts and ground linseeds. Cover and leave overnight in the fridge. Serve in individual bowls, topped with the fresh berries.

HEALTH STATISTICS

Oats are rich in soluble fibre, which helps regulate blood sugar and insulin levels as well as reduce cholesterol levels. They also supply B vitamins, iron, magnesium and zinc. The nuts supply vitamin E, essential fatty acids and protein. Brazils are particularly good for selenium while walnuts and linseeds are excellent sources of omega-3 oils. The berries give you a great boost of vitamin C and cancer-protective phytonutrients.

NUTRITIONAL ANALYSIS (PER SERVING):

Calories 364 kcal	Carbohydrate 49 g
Protein 12 g	Total sugars* 17 g
Fat 15 g	Fibre 5.6 g
Saturates 2.4 g	Salt 0.1 g

* total sugars includes sugars found naturally in foods

BIO-YOGHURT WITH BANANA AND HONEY

MAKES 2 SERVINGS

I can't help thinking that honey and fruit together are such a decadent combination, so what better (and a more nutritious) way to start the day than adding some live bio-yoghurt and toasted nuts. A real superfood fix!

2 ripe bananas
300 g (10 oz) plain live bio-yoghurt
1–2 level tablespoons (15–30 ml) honey
2 tablespoons toasted flaked almonds (or walnuts, hazelnuts or pecans)

▸ Slice the bananas into two bowls. Spoon half the yoghurt on top of each bowl. Drizzle with honey and scatter over the toasted nuts.

HEALTH STATISTICS

Live bio-yoghurt contains health-boosting lactobacillus and bifida bacteria, which promote healthy digestion, help reduce bloating and boost your immune system. It's also a great source of protein and bone-strengthening calcium. Bananas supply fibre, potassium and vitamin B6 while the nuts add vitamin E and essential fatty acids.

NUTRITIONAL ANALYSIS (PER SERVING):

Calories 309kcal	Carbohydrate 48g
Protein 11g	Total sugars* 45g
Fat 9.2g	Fibre 2.1g
Saturates 1.7g	Salt 0.2g

* total sugars includes sugars found naturally in foods

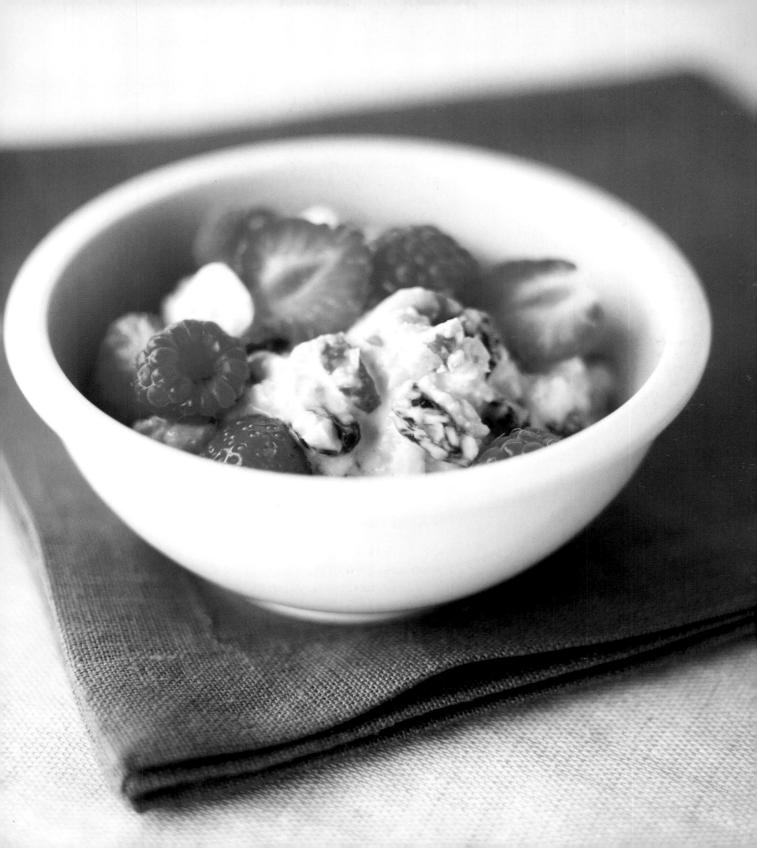

CHAPTER 5
BEANS AND LENTILS

HUMMUS WITH PINE NUTS

MAKES 4 SERVINGS

This rustic version of hummus contains whole chickpeas and combines
beautifully with the toasted pine nuts. Serve with olives, cherry tomatoes,
carrot, cucumber and pepper strips, or spread on rye crackers or rice cakes
for a delicious nourishing lunch. It will keep in the fridge for up to 3 days

400 g (14 oz) tinned chickpeas or
125 g (4 oz) dried chickpeas, soaked overnight
then boiled for 45 minutes
1–2 garlic cloves, crushed
2 tablespoons (30 ml) extra virgin olive oil
1 tablespoon (15 ml) tahini (sesame seed paste)
Juice of ½ lemon
2–4 tablespoons (30–60 ml) water
A little low-sodium salt and freshly ground black pepper
1–2 tablespoons (15–30 ml) pine nuts

▸ Drain and rinse the chickpeas. Reserve 1–2 tablespoons of chickpeas. Put the
remainder in a food processor or blender with the garlic, olive oil, tahini, lemon juice
and water. Whizz until smooth, add a little low-sodium salt and freshly ground black
pepper and process again. Taste to check the seasoning. Add extra water if necessary
to give the desired consistency.

▸ Meanwhile, toast the pine nuts under a hot grill for 3–4 minutes until they are lightly
coloured but not brown (watch carefully as they colour quickly).

▸ Stir the reserved whole chickpeas into the mixture. Spoon into a shallow dish. Scatter
over the pine nuts and drizzle over a few drops of olive oil. Chill in the fridge for at least
two hours before serving.

HEALTH STATISTICS
Chickpeas provide lots of fibre, protein and
iron. They also contain fructo-oligosaccharides,
a type of fibre that boosts the friendly bacteria
of the gut and benefits the immune system. Pine
nuts are rich in heart-protective vitamin E, zinc
and iron.

NUTRITIONAL ANALYSIS (PER SERVING):

Calories 219 kcal	Carbohydrate 16 g
Protein 8.6 g	Total sugars* 0.6 g
Fat 14 g	Fibre 4.6 g
Saturates 1.7 g	Salt 0.5 g **

* total sugars includes sugars found naturally in foods
**the salt content will be lower if you rinse the beans well
or use beans tinned in water rather than salted water

BUTTER BEAN DIP

MAKES 4 SERVINGS

This dip is also perfect served with crudités, such as carrot, cucumber, celery and red pepper strips, as well as as a spread for toast. Keep any remainder covered in the fridge for up to three days

400 g (14 oz) tin butter beans
1 garlic clove, crushed
Juice of 1/2 lemon
2 tablespoons (30 ml) olive oil
A little low-sodium salt and freshly ground black pepper
1 tablespoon (15 ml) chopped fresh parsley

▸ Drain and rinse the butter beans. Put in a food processor or blender with the garlic, lemon juice, and olive oil. Whizz until smooth, add a little low-sodium salt and freshly ground black pepper and process again. Add a little water if it's too thick.
▸ Stir in the parsley. Spoon into a shallow dish and chill in the fridge before serving.

HEALTH STATISTICS

Butter beans are rich in protein and complex carbohydrates. They have a low glycaemic index and release their energy over a long period of time so you feel satisfied longer. They're also an excellent source of potassium, which helps regulate fluid levels in the body and control blood pressure, as well as calcium, magnesium, iron and B vitamins.

NUTRITIONAL ANALYSIS (PER SERVING):

Calories 126 kcal	Carbohydrate 13 g
Protein 5.9 g	Total sugars* 1.1 g
Fat 6.0 g	Fibre 4.6 g
Saturates 0.9 g	Salt 1.0 g**

* total sugars includes sugars found naturally in foods
** the salt content will be lower if you rinse the beans well or use beans tinned in water rather than salted water

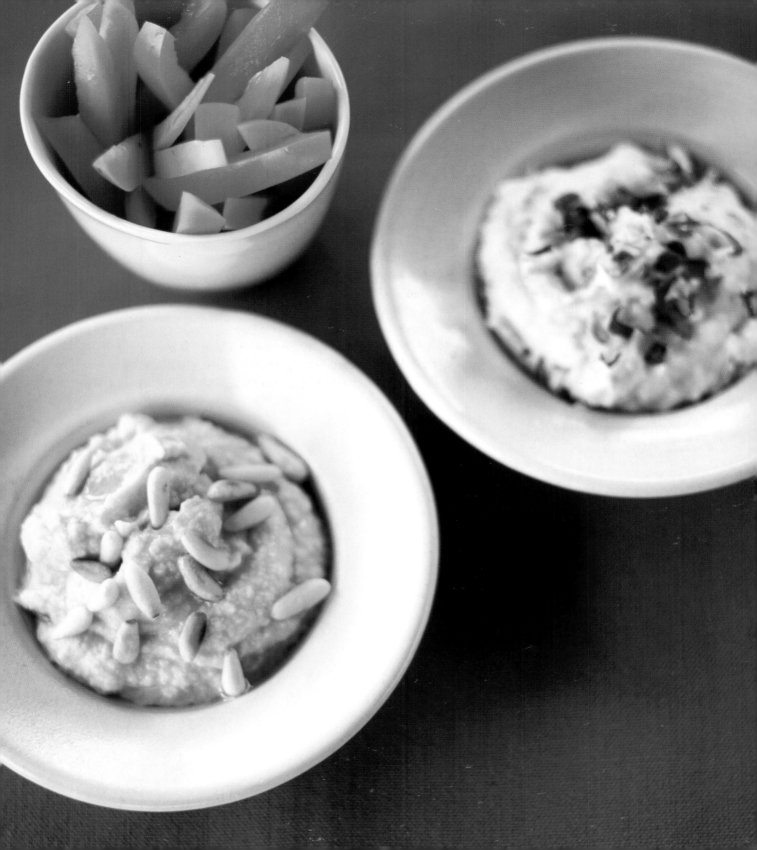

TUNA ON LENTILS AND MUSHROOMS

MAKES 2 SERVINGS

This fashionable way of serving fresh fish not only looks and tastes amazing but is surprisingly simple.

400 g (14 oz) can brown lentils, drained
400 g (14 oz) can cherry tomatoes
125 g (4 oz) button mushrooms
125 g (4 oz) fresh tomatoes, halved or quartered
2 x 150 g tuna steaks
Small handful fresh basil leaves

► Mix the canned lentils, mushrooms and fresh tomatoes in a saucepan. Bring to the boil, reduce the heat and simmer for ten minutes until slightly thickened.
► Brush the tuna steaks with a little olive oil. Heat a non-stick pan until hot. Add the tuna and fry for 2–3 minutes, turn over and cook the other side for 3 minutes. Remove from heat.
► Divide the lentil mixture onto two plates, scatter over the basil, then lay a tuna steak on top.

HEALTH STATISTICS

Brown lentils are an excellent source of fibre, which helps promote a healthy digestive system, reduce transit time and reduce cholesterol levels in the blood. They also supply protein, iron and magnesium. Fresh tuna (but not the tinned version) is rich in omega-3 oils, which helps prevent heart attacks and stroke, and alleviate inflammatory conditions such as arthritis.

NUTRITIONAL ANALYSIS (PER SERVING):

Calories 433 kcal	Carbohydrate 36 g
Protein 55 g	Total sugars* 2.9 g
Fat 8. 8g	Fibre 8.9 g
Saturates 2.1 g	Salt 1.1 g**

* total sugars includes sugars found naturally in foods
** the salt content will be lower if you rinse the lentils well or use dried lentils boiled in unsalted water

BORLOTTI BEAN AND TOMATO HOTPOT

MAKES 2 SERVINGS

Borlotti beans look quite dull on their own, so it's important to combine them with bright coloured ingredients as in this simple recipe. Serve this dish with basmati or brown rice an extra green vegetable.

1 tablespoon (15 ml) olive oil
1 onion, sliced
1 garlic clove, crushed
1 yellow pepper, deseeded and diced
1 red pepper, deseeded and diced
200g (7 oz) tin chopped tomatoes
200g (½ tin) borlotti beans, drained
1 teaspoon (5 ml) vegetable bouillon

▸ Heat the olive oil in a large non-stick pan. Add the onion, garlic and peppers and sauté for about 5 minutes until the vegetables have softened.
▸ Add the tomatoes, beans and bouillon, stir and bring to the boil. Simmer for 15–20 minutes until the vegetables are tender, the flavours have infused nicely and the sauce has reduced a little.

HEALTH STATISTICS
This recipe is brimful of vitamin C and beta-carotene from the colourful peppers. The vitamins are kept in the dish as the cooking liquid is not discarded. It also provides lycopene – a powerful anti-cancer nutrient – from the tomatoes as well as fibre and protein from the beans.

NUTRITIONAL ANALYSIS (PER SERVING):

Calories 216 kcal	Carbohydrate 31 g
Protein 9.6 g	Total sugars* 17 g
Fat 6.7 g	Fibre 9.0 g
Saturates 1.0 g	Salt 1.2 g**

* total sugars includes sugars found naturally in foods
** the salt content will be lower if you rinse the beans well or use beans tinned in water rather than salted water

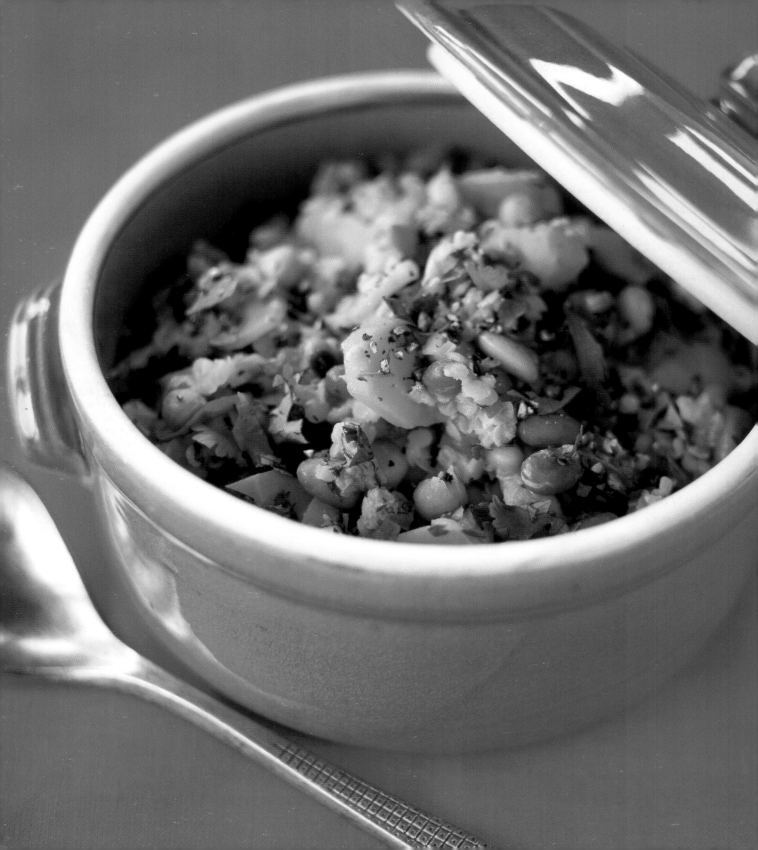

MIXED BEAN AND LENTIL HOTPOT WITH FRESH CORIANDER

MAKES 2 SERVINGS

Keep your store cupboard stocked with tinned beans and dried lentils and you'll always have an easy meal at hand. This recipe combines both of these nutritious ingredients with a few colourful vegetables.

1 tablespoon (15 ml) olive or rapeseed oil
1 onion, chopped
1 small red pepper, diced
1 garlic clove, crushed
125 g (4 oz) red lentils
500 ml (16 fl oz) vegetable stock
2 carrots, sliced
200 g (½ tin) mixed beans in water, rinsed and drained
1 tablespoon (15 ml) lemon juice
A little low-sodium salt
A small handful of fresh coriander, finely chopped

▸ Heat the oil in a heavy based pan and sauté the onions for 5 minutes. Add the garlic and red pepper and continue cooking for 1 minute while stirring continuously.
▸ Add the lentils, stock, carrots and beans. Bring to the boil. Cover and simmer for about 25 minutes, then season with the lemon juice and low-sodium salt. Finally, stir in the fresh coriander.
▸ Serve with cooked quinoa or brown rice and a spoonful of low-fat natural yoghurt.

HEALTH STATISTICS
Red lentils and beans are highly nutritious foods: they provide a good balance of protein and complex carbohydrates as well as soluble fibre, iron, B vitamins, zinc and magnesium. This dish has a low glycaemic index, which means it will give you long-lasting energy and keep you feeling satisfied longer.

NUTRITIONAL ANALYSIS (PER SERVING):

Calories 416 kcal	Carbohydrate 68 g
Protein 24 g	Total sugars* 18 g
Fat 7.5 g	Fibre 13 g
Saturates 1.3 g	Salt 1.1 g**

* total sugars includes sugars found naturally in foods
** the salt content will be lower if you rinse the beans well, or use beans tinned in water rather than salted water

CHICKPEA AND FLAGEOLET BEAN BURGERS WITH TOMATO SALSA

MAKES 8

This is one of my favourite vegetarian burger recipes that I use to convince sceptical meat-eating guests at barbecues that you can create delicious al fresco food without meat!

400 g (14 oz) can chickpeas, rinsed and drained
400 g (14 oz) can flageolet beans, rinsed and drained
1 small onion, finely chopped
1 teaspoon (5 ml) curry powder
1 tablespoon (15 ml) chopped parsley
25 g (1 oz) fresh breadcrumbs
1 egg

FOR THE TOMATO SALSA:
2 large ripe tomatoes
½ small red onion, finely chopped
1 celery stick, finely chopped
Small handful fresh coriander, chopped
1 small clove of garlic, crushed
1 tbsp (15 ml) olive oil
2 tbsp (30 ml) lemon or lime juice

▸ Put the drained chickpeas, beans, onion, curry powder, parsley, breadcrumbs and egg in a bowl and mix together using a large fork. Alternatively, place in a food processor and process until combined.

▸ Preheat the grill.

▸ Divide the mixture into eight, form into balls and press down to form burger shapes.

▸ Place the burgers on an oiled baking tray then brush with olive oil and grill for 4 minutes on each side until golden brown.

▸ Mix together the salsa ingredients. Serve with a green salad.

HEALTH STATISTICS
These highly nutritious burgers are excellent sources of protein and fibre. They'll also give you lots of iron and B vitamins. The fresh salsa contains immune-enhancing vitamin C and cancer-protective lycopene. Fresh coriander is a great source of iron.

NUTRITIONAL ANALYSIS (PER BURGER):

Calories 151 kcal	Carbohydrate 21 g
Protein 8.7 g	Total sugars* 3.3 g
Fat 4.1 g	Fibre 6.0 g
Saturates 0.7 g	Salt 0.4 g**

* total sugars includes sugars found naturally in foods
** the salt content will be lower if you rinse the beans well or use beans tinned in water rather than salted water

DAHL WITH SWEET POTATOES AND COCONUT

MAKES 2 SERVINGS

I love this lightly spiced dish. You can add other vegetables, such as cauliflower florets, button mushrooms or broccoli, if you wish.

1 onion, chopped
85g (3oz) red lentils
200 ml (7 fl oz) coconut milk
225 ml (8 fl oz) water
1 sweet potato (weighing approx 250 g/9 oz), cut into small pieces
1–2 garlic cloves, crushed
½ teaspoon (2.5 ml) fresh grated ginger
½ teaspoon (2.5 ml) ground cumin
1 teaspoon (5 ml) ground coriander
½ teaspoon (1.25 ml) turmeric
A little low-sodium salt and freshly ground black pepper
Handful of fresh coriander or parsley, finely chopped

▸ Put the onion, lentils, coconut milk, water, sweet potato and garlic in a large saucepan.
▸ Bring to the boil, then lower the heat and simmer gently for 20 minutes until the lentils and sweet potatoes are tender. The dhal will be quite thick, like porridge.
▸ Stir in the ginger, spices, low-sodium salt and pepper and cook for a few more minutes. Stir in the coriander.
▸ Serve with steamed green cabbage or broccoli.

HEALTH STATISTICS
Red lentils have a low glycaemic index, which means you feel full of energy for a long time and won't get hungry between meals. They are a great source of protein, fibre, iron and B vitamins. The sweet potato provides good amounts of beta-carotene, useful for helping protect against cancer and heart disease.

NUTRITIONAL ANALYSIS (PER SERVING):

Calories 293 kcal	Carbohydrate 61 g
Protein 13 g	Total sugars* 17 g
Fat 1.4 g	Fibre 6.1 g
Saturates 0.4 g	Salt 0.5 g

* total sugars includes sugars found naturally in foods

BEAN AND SPINACH BURGERS

MAKES 8

This recipe is made from store cupboard standbys – tinned beans and sweetcorn – and frozen spinach. If you don't need all the burgers for one meal, you can freeze the remainder for another occasion.

1 tablespoon (15 ml) olive oil
1 small red onion, finely chopped
1 garlic clove, crushed
1 small red chilli, deseeded (optional)
2 x 400 g (14 oz) tins borlotti beans, drained
198 g (7 oz) tin sweetcorn, drained
400 g frozen chopped spinach, thawed
60 g (2 oz) fresh wholemeal breadcrumbs
1 teaspoon (5 ml) ground cumin
1 tablespoon (15 ml) chopped fresh coriander

▸ Pre-heat the oven to 190°C/375°F/Gas mark 5.
▸ Heat the oil in a non-stick frying pan. Add the onions, garlic and chilli and cook over a moderate heat for 3 minutes until softened but not browned.
▸ Place the beans, sweetcorn, spinach, breadcrumbs, cumin and coriander in a large mixing bowl. Add the onion mixture and mash together until well combined. Shape the mixture into 8 burgers.
▸ Place the burgers on an oiled baking tray and brush with olive oil. Bake in the oven for 25–30 minutes until they are lightly browned and crisp on the outside.
▸ Serve with a leafy salad.

HEALTH STATISTICS
Unlike the meat version, these vegetarian burgers are rich in fibre. Borlotti beans are also good sources of protein, iron and zinc, while the spinach adds folate, iron, calcium and vitamin C.

NUTRITIONAL ANALYSIS (PER BURGER):

Calories 149 kcal	Carbohydrate 24 g
Protein 9.0 g	Total sugars* 4.3 g
Fat 2.8 g	Fibre 6.5 g
Saturates 0.4 g	Salt 1.3 g**

* total sugars includes sugars found naturally in foods
** the salt content will be lower if you rinse the beans well or use beans tinned in water rather than salted water

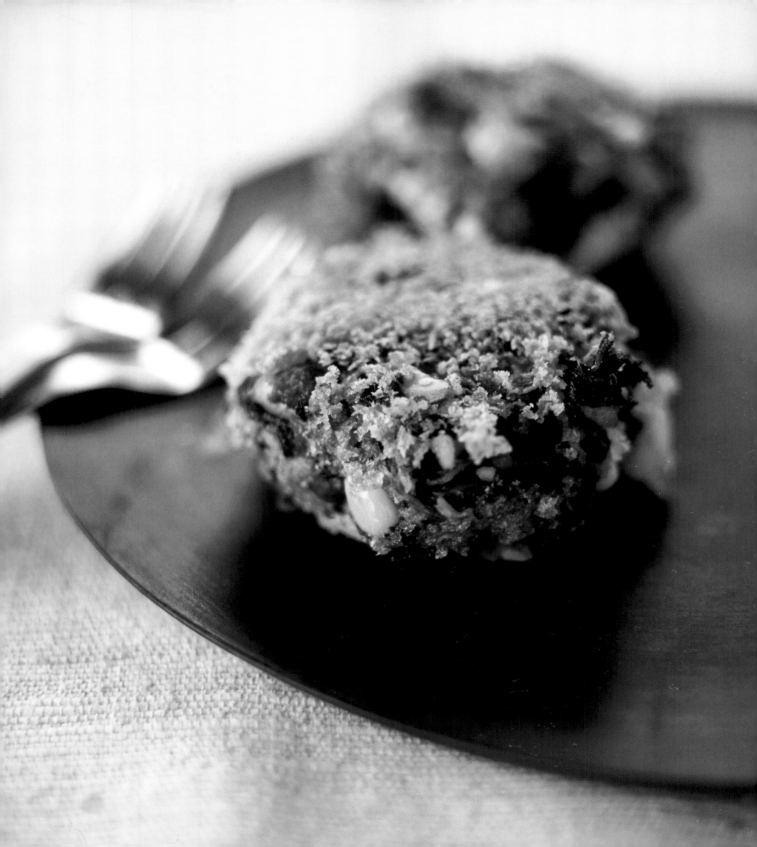

CHICKPEAS WITH MUSHROOMS AND SPINACH

MAKES 2 SERVINGS

This hearty hot pot is an interesting combination of colours, textures and flavours. I love the delicate slightly nutty flavour of chickpeas, which work really well with earthy shitake mushrooms and vibrant spinach. If you can't get shitake mushrooms, use any other variety.

1 tablespoon (15 ml) extra virgin olive oil
1 onion, chopped
1 garlic clove, crushed
$1/2$ red pepper, deseeded and chopped
60 g (2 oz) shitake mushrooms, sliced
4 tomatoes, skinned and chopped
250 ml (8 fl oz) vegetable stock
400 g (14 oz) tinned chickpeas, drained and rinsed
125 g (4 oz) fresh spinach, washed and trimmed

▸ Heat the oil in a heavy based pan, add the onion, garlic and red pepper and cook over a moderate heat for 5 minutes.

▸ Add the mushrooms, tomatoes, vegetable stock and chickpeas. Stir, then bring to the boil. Lower the heat and simmer for 20 minutes, stirring occasionally.

▸ Stir in the spinach, cover and continue cooking for 2–3 minutes until the spinach is wilted. Serve in individual bowls.

HEALTH STATISTICS
Chickpeas are powerhouses of nutrients, providing a near-perfect balance of complex carbohydrates and protein, as well as B vitamins, fibre, iron and zinc. The spinach in this recipe is a great source of iron, folate and beta-carotene, while the red peppers and tomatoes provide plenty of vitamin C.

NUTRITIONAL ANALYSIS (PER SERVING):

Calories 380 kcal	Carbohydrate 51 g
Protein 19 g	Total sugars* 14 g
Fat 13 g	Fibre 13 g
Saturates 1.7 g	Salt 1.4 g**

* total sugars includes sugars found naturally in foods
** the salt content will be lower if you rinse the beans well or use beans tinned in water rather than salted water

RED KIDNEY BEAN TAGINE WITH BULGAR WHEAT

MAKES 2 SERVINGS

This mildly spiced Moroccan-inspired dish can be made in advance which also gives the flavours blend and improve. You can make a larger quantity and keep the remainder in the fridge for up to 3 days or the freezer for up to 3 months.

1 tablespoon (15 ml) olive oil
1 onion, sliced
1 garlic clove, crushed
½ teaspoon (2.5 ml) turmeric
½ teaspoon (2.5 ml) ground ginger
1 red pepper, deseeded and diced
1 courgette, sliced thickly
½ small aubergine, diced
200g (7 oz) tin chopped tomatoes

200g (½ tin) red kidney beans, drained
60 g (2 oz) black olives, pitted
150 ml (5 fl oz) vegetable stock
85 g (3 oz) bulgar (cracked) wheat
A little low-sodium salt
Freshly ground black pepper
Small handful of coriander leaves, roughly chopped

▸ Heat the olive oil in a large non-stick pan. Add the onions and cook gently for 10 minutes, stirring occasionally. Add the garlic, turmeric and ginger and stir for a few moments. Add the pepper, courgette and aubergine and continue cooking for a few minutes, then add the tomatoes, beans, olives and vegetable stock. Stir and bring to the boil. Cover and simmer for 15 minutes or until the vegetables are tender.
▸ While the tagine is cooking, put the bulgar wheat in a bowl and add lukewarm water until just covered. Leave for 15 minutes, drain, then transfer back to the bowl. Fluff with a fork, season with the low-sodium salt and freshly ground black pepper, and then stir in the coriander. Serve with the tagine.

HEALTH STATISTICS
Red kidney beans are an excellent source of fibre which promotes a healthy balance of friendly bacteria in the gut, thus improving your health and immunity. They also supply protein, which complement the cereal protein provided by the bulgar wheat. The overall quality of the protein is therefore enhanced. This dish also supplies zinc, iron and selenium

NUTRITIONAL ANALYSIS (PER SERVING):

Calories 415 kcal	Carbohydrate 66 g
Protein 15 g	Total sugars* 17 g
Fat 11 g	Fibre 12 g
Saturates 1.6 g	Salt 1.1 g

* total sugars includes sugars found naturally in foods
** the salt content will be lower if you rinse the beans well or use beans tinned in water rather than salted water or use olives in olive oil rather than brine

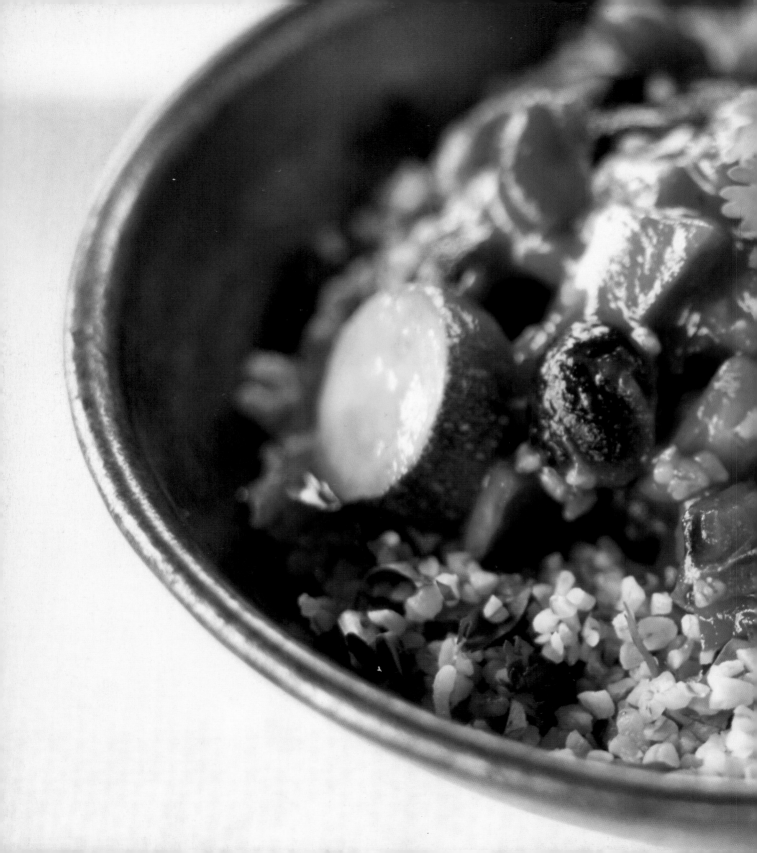

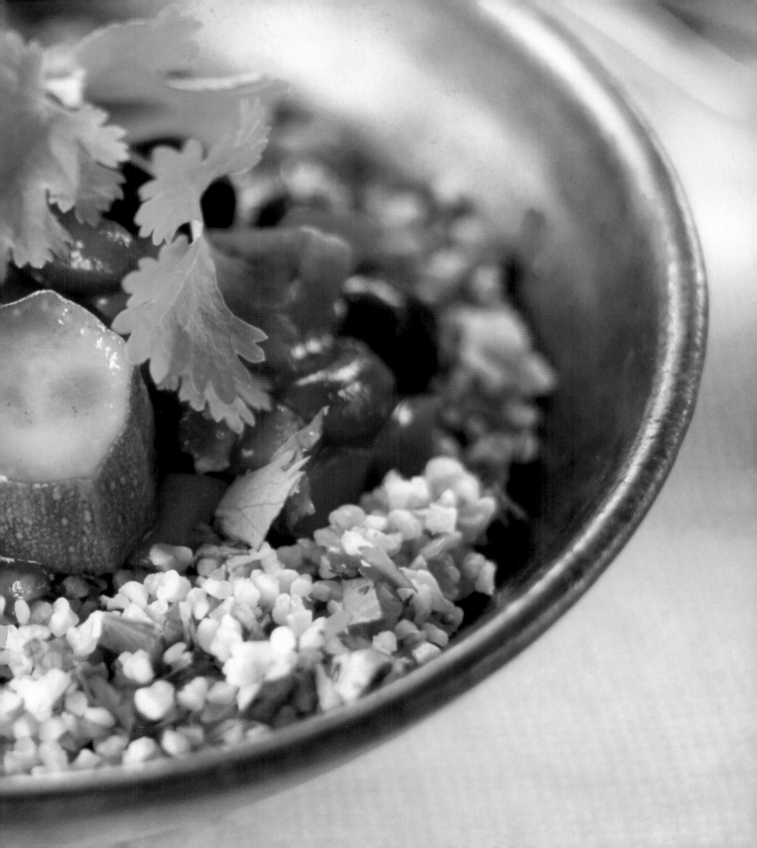

CHAPTER 6
GRAINS

SPICED RICE WITH CHICKPEAS AND OLIVES

MAKES 2 SERVINGS

If you've often wondered what to do with a can of chickpeas, here is an easy and tasty recipe that combines the nutritional benefits of chickpeas and wholegrain rice.

1 tablespoon (15 ml) olive oil
1 onion, finely chopped
1 garlic clove, crushed
1 teaspoon (5 ml) ground coriander
½ teaspoon (2.5 ml) cumin seeds
60 g button mushrooms
1 courgette, trimmed and sliced
1 x 425 g can chickpeas, drained
125 g (4 oz) brown rice
400 ml (14 fl oz) vegetable stock
60 g (2 oz) black olives (pitted)
Small handful of fresh coriander, roughly chopped
A little low-sodium salt and freshly ground black pepper

▸ Heat the oil in a large heavy based pan. Add the onion and cook over a moderate heat for 5 minutes until softened. Add the garlic, coriander, cumin seeds, mushrooms and courgettes and cook for two minutes.

▸ Stir in the chickpeas, brown rice and vegetable stock then bring to the boil. Cover, reduce the heat and simmer for 20–25 minutes until the liquid has been absorbed and the rice is cooked. Add the olives and chopped coriander, season with the low-sodium salt and pepper and serve.

HEALTH STATISTICS
Wholegrain (brown) rice has a lower glycaemic index (GI) than the white variety so will give you longer lasting energy and prevent hunger pangs. It also provides fibre, magnesium, phosphorus, thiamin (vitamin B1) and iron, as well as some protein. Combining brown rice with chickpeas boosts the overall protein quality of the meal. You'll also get fibre, iron and B vitamins from the chickpeas and vitamin E from the olives.

NUTRITIONAL ANALYSIS (PER SERVING):

Calories 553 kcal	Carbohydrate 90 g
Protein 21 g	Total sugars* 6.7 g
Fat 15 g	Fibre 12 g
Saturates 2.1 g	Salt 1.7 g**

* total sugars includes sugars found naturally in foods
** This figure will be lower if you rinse the olives or use olives in olive oil rather than brine

PAN FRIED SALMON ON CANNELLINI BEANS WITH SOBA NOODLES

MAKES 1 SERVING

You can barbecue or grill the fish if you like – just make the beans in advance.

1 tablespoon (15 ml) olive oil
1 garlic clove, crushed
125 g (4 oz) tinned cannellini beans, drained
60 g (2 oz) cherry tomatoes
Juice and zest of ½ lemon
150 g (5 oz) salmon fillet
A handful of rocket
60 g (2 oz) soba (buckwheat) noodles
A drizzle of sesame oil

▸ Heat the olive oil in a non-stick frying pan and cook the garlic for 1 minute.
Add the beans, tomatoes and lemon juice. Warm over a low heat for 5 minutes.
▸ Brush the salmon fillet with a little olive oil. Heat a non-stick pan until hot. Add the salmon and fry for 4–5 minutes, turn it over and cook the other side for 3 minutes. Remove from heat.
▸ Bring a large pan of water to the boil, add the noodles and cook for 2 minutes.
Drain and rinse under cold running water. Transfer to a bowl, sprinkle with the sesame oil and stir briefly to coat.
▸ Pile the soba noodles and then the beans onto a serving plate, scatter over the rocket.
Place the salmon on top and serve immediately.

HEALTH STATISTICS
Salmon is rich in omega-3 oils, which help prevent strokes and heart attacks, as well as improving blood flow and oxygen delivery to your cells. (including around the cellulite areas). Soba noodles – made from buckwheat flour – have a low GI and also supply good amounts of magnesium and iron

NUTRITIONAL ANALYSIS (PER SERVING):

Calories 600 kcal	Carbohydrate 52 g
Protein 43 g	Total sugars* 6.6 g
Fat 26 g	Fibre 8.4 g
Saturates 3.9 g	Salt 1.2 g

* total sugars includes sugars found naturally in foods

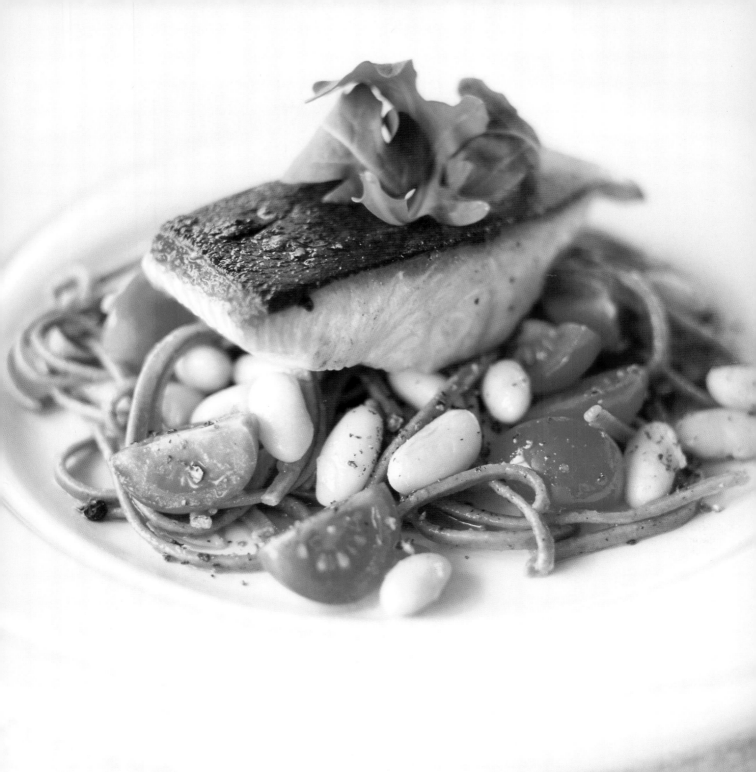

CHICKEN WITH VERMICELLI NOODLES AND CORIANDER

MAKES 1 SERVING

This Malaysian inspired recipe is a delicious and healthy way of serving chicken. Use other raw vegetables such as grated carrots or courgettes if you wish.

½ red pepper
15 cm (6 in) cucumber
2 spring onions
1 tablespoon (15 ml) lime juice
60 g (2 oz) rice vermicelli noodles
1 cooked chicken breast
A drizzle of sesame oil
A small handful of fresh coriander, roughly chopped
1 tablespoon (15 ml) peanuts, roughly chopped

▸ Slice the red pepper thinly and cut the cucumber into thin strips. Chop the spring onions into small pieces. Place the prepared vegetables in a bowl, add the lime juice and toss well.

▸ Pour boiling water over the noodles and leave to soak for 6 minutes. Drain, then rinse in cold water and drain again.

▸ Roughly shred the cooked chicken. Add to the vegetables along with the noodles and coriander leaves. Sprinkle over a little sesame oil and toss lightly. Scatter with the peanuts and serve.

HEALTH STATISTICS
This dish provides a good balance of protein and carbohydrate. Chicken supplies B vitamins and contains a low level of fat. The red pepper, lime juice and coriander are all excellent providers of vitamin C, which can help boost collagen production.

NUTRITIONAL ANALYSIS (PER SERVING):

Calories 472 kcal	Carbohydrate 54 g
Protein 40 g	Total sugars* 7.5 g
Fat 12 g	Fibre 4.1 g
Saturates 1.8 g	Salt 0.1 g

* total sugars includes sugars found naturally in foods

MOROCCAN CHICKEN WITH QUINOA

MAKES 1 SERVING

This mildly spiced dish is a delicious way of cooking chicken. It needs marinating for at least 30 minutes, so remember to plan ahead.

1 skinless chicken breast
1 garlic clove, crushed
½ red chilli, deseeded and chopped (use according to taste)
A pinch of paprika
A pinch of ground cumin
1 lemon
1 tablespoon (15 ml) fresh mint leaves
60 g (2 oz) quinoa (or brown rice)
1 tablespoon (15 ml) toasted pumpkin seeds

▸ Slash the chicken breast 3 or 4 times.
▸ Place the garlic, chilli, paprika, cumin, the juice of half the lemon and mint leaves in a bowl and mix well. Add the chicken and turn a few times. Leave to marinate for at least 30 minutes.
▸ Meanwhile, boil the quinoa (or rice) according to packet instructions (approximately 25 minutes). Drain and mix with the toasted pumpkin seeds.
▸ Pre-heat the grill. Place the chicken on a baking tray and grill for 6 or 7 minutes each side until cooked through.
▸ Spoon the quinoa on a plate and place the chicken on top. Serve with a green vegetable.

HEALTH STATISTICS
Quinoa is available from health food stores and health food sections of larger supermarkets. Strictly, a fruit rather than a grain, it contains higher levels of protein than grains as well as good amounts of fibre, B vitamins, vitamin E and zinc.

NUTRITIONAL ANALYSIS (PER SERVING):

Calories 431 kcal	Carbohydrate 37 g
Protein 42 g	Total sugars* 4.0 g
Fat 14 g	Fibre 0.6 g
Saturates 2.3 g	Salt 0.3 g

* total sugars includes sugars found naturally in foods

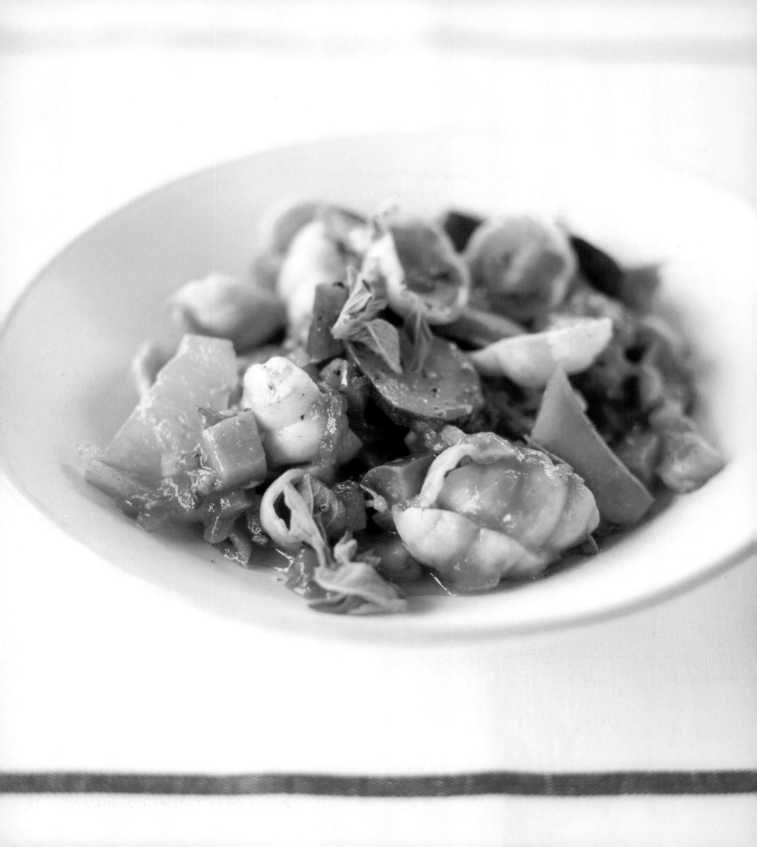

PASTA SHELLS WITH CHUNKY VEGETABLE SAUCE

MAKES 2 SERVINGS

This delicious chunky tomato-based sauce can be varied with lots of different vegetables. Try adding diced root vegetables such as sweet potato, swede, and carrot or even butternut squash and pumpkin.

2 tablespoons (30 ml) extra virgin olive oil
1 onion, peeled and chopped
1 yellow pepper, deseeded and chopped
1 garlic clove, crushed
4 button mushrooms, wiped and cut in half
1 small courgette, sliced
½ aubergine, diced
60 g (2oz) mange tout, trimmed and cut in half
400 g (14 oz) can tomatoes
1 teaspoon (5ml) oregano
A little low-sodium salt and freshly ground black pepper
175 g (6 oz) wholewheat or non-wheat pasta shells

▸ Heat the oil in a large saucepan. Cook the onion and pepper for 5 minutes. Add the garlic, mushrooms, courgettes, aubergine, mange tout and tinned tomatoes. Stir to mix well, then bring to the boil, cover and simmer for about 20 minutes until the vegetables are tender. Add the oregano and season to taste with low-sodium salt and freshly ground black pepper.
▸ Meanwhile, cook the pasta in boiling water according to the packet instructions. Drain, then add to the vegetable sauce, stir well and serve.

HEALTH STATISTICS

This sauce is packed with fibre and antioxidant vitamins, including vitamin C from the peppers and mange tout. Tinned tomatoes are rich in lycopene, which helps protect against prostate and breast cancer and guard against heart attacks. Lycopene is absorbed more readily from cooked tomatoes than fresh, which makes this sauce an excellent way of boosting your lycopene quota.

NUTRITIONAL ANALYSIS (PER SERVING):

Calories 509 kcal	Carbohydrate 86 g
Protein 17 g	Total sugars* 19 g
Fat 14 g	Fibre 8.6 g
Saturates 1.9 g	Salt 0.24 g

* total sugars includes sugars found naturally in foods

PASTA AND BEAN SALAD WITH GRAPES AND BLACK OLIVES

MAKES 2 SERVINGS

I love making this salad with different kinds of beans. It's also good with flageolet beans, borlotti beans and black-eye beans. On colder days, omit the dressing and grapes, add the beans and vegetables to the drained pasta in a saucepan and warm through.

125 g (4 oz) wholewheat or non-wheat pasta shapes
125 g (4 oz) tinned red kidney beans, rinsed and drained
125 g (4 oz) tinned chickpeas, rinsed and drained
85 g (3 oz) cherry tomatoes, halved
85 g (3 oz) red grapes
60 g (2 oz) stoned black olives
1 tablespoon (15 ml) fresh mint, roughly chopped
1 tablespoon (15 ml) fresh flat leaf parsley

FOR THE DRESSING:
2 tablespoons (30 ml) olive oil;
1 tablespoon (15 ml) lemon juice
1 teaspoon (5 ml) balsamic vinegar
Freshly ground black pepper

▸ Cook the pasta according to packet instructions. Drain, then transfer to a large bowl.
▸ Add the beans, chickpeas, tomatoes, grapes, olives, mint and parsley. Mix to combine.
▸ For the dressing: place the olive oil, lemon juice and balsamic vinegar in a bottle or screw-top jar and shake together thoroughly. Pour over the salad then toss gently. Season with freshly ground black pepper.

HEALTH STATISTICS
The different proteins in the beans and pasta complement each other so you end up with an excellent balance of protein that's also low in fat and very filling. Beans provide soluble fibre, which not only slows the absorption of carbohydrates from the intestines but also helps lower blood cholesterol levels. The salad also provides vitamins A, C and E, and healthy monounsaturated oils.

NUTRITIONAL ANALYSIS (PER SERVING):

Calories 343 kcal	Carbohydrate 40 g
Protein 11 g	Total sugars* 10 g
Fat 16 g	Fibre 9.6 g
Saturates 2.3 g	Salt 1.2 g**

* total sugars includes sugars found naturally in foods
** This figure will be lower if you rinse the beans and olives well

SPAGHETTI WITH FRESH TOMATOES AND BASIL

MAKES 2 SERVINGS

Make this simple dish in the summer when fresh tomatoes are plentiful and full of flavour. Serve with a leafy salad.

4 medium vine ripened tomatoes
175 g (6 oz) wholewheat or non-wheat spaghetti
A small handful fresh basil leaves
2 tablespoons (30 ml) extra virgin olive oil
A little low-sodium salt and freshly ground black pepper
25 g (1 oz) pine nuts, lightly toasted

▸ Skin the tomatoes. Place in a bowl and pour over boiling water, leave for one minute, and then drain off the water. Pierce the skin with a sharp knife and the skin should slide off quite easily. Chop the tomatoes roughly.

▸ Cook the pasta in boiling water according to the packet instructions. Drain, then return to the saucepan. Add the chopped tomatoes, roughly torn basil leaves, olive oil and seasoning. Stir well to mix over a gentle heat for a minute to warm through. Divide between two bowls and scatter over the pine nuts.

HEALTH STATISTICS
Fresh tomatoes are rich in immune-boosting vitamin C – this recipe supplies 27 mg vitamin C, approximately 70 per cent of your daily needs. Vitamin C helps strengthen collagen and thus improve the appearance of cellulite. They also provide good amounts of vitamin E and potassium. Fresh basil supplies extra beta-carotene and iron.

NUTRITIONAL ANALYSIS (PER SERVING):

Calories 431 kcal	Carbohydrate 53 g
Protein 10 g	Total sugars* 7.1 g
Fat 21 g	Fibre 7.1 g
Saturates 2.5 g	Salt 0.1 g

* total sugars includes sugars found naturally in foods

SPICED QUINOA PILAFF

MAKES 2 SERVINGS

This is one of my favourite ways of serving quinoa. It's very easy to make as everything is cooked in one pan. You can add other vegetables, such as peas and green beans, and a handful of toasted cashews or walnuts.

1 tablespoon (15 ml) extra virgin olive oil
1 small onion, chopped
1 garlic clove, crushed
1 teaspoon (5 ml) cumin seeds
½ teaspoon (2.5 ml) turmeric
1 red pepper, deseeded and chopped
125 g (4 oz) quinoa
600 ml (1 pint) vegetable stock
2 tablespoons (30 ml) sultanas
A little low-sodium salt and freshly ground black pepper
Handful of fresh coriander leaves, roughly chopped

▸ Heat the oil in a large saucepan and sauté the onion over a gentle heat for 5 minutes.
▸ Add the garlic, cumin seeds, turmeric and pepper and continue cooking for 3 minutes.
▸ Add the quinoa and vegetable stock, stir well, then bring to the boil. Reduce the heat and simmer for about 20 minutes until the liquid has been absorbed and the grains are tender.
▸ Season with low-sodium salt and black pepper. Stir in the sultanas and coriander.
▸ Serve with lightly steamed vegetables and grilled fish, chicken or tofu.

HEALTH STATISTICS

Quinoa has a low glycaemic index so will make you feel satisfied for longer, prevent hunger and keep your blood sugar levels steady. It provides a good source of protein, magnesium, zinc, fibre and vitamin E. The pepper provides plenty of vitamin C, which is good for strengthening collagen and the walls of your small blood vessels.

NUTRITIONAL ANALYSIS (PER SERVING):

Calories 328 kcal	Carbohydrate 55 g
Protein 16 g	Total sugars* 23 g
Fat 9.1 g	Fibre 2.1 g
Saturates 1.2 g	Salt 0.1 g

* total sugars includes sugars found naturally in foods

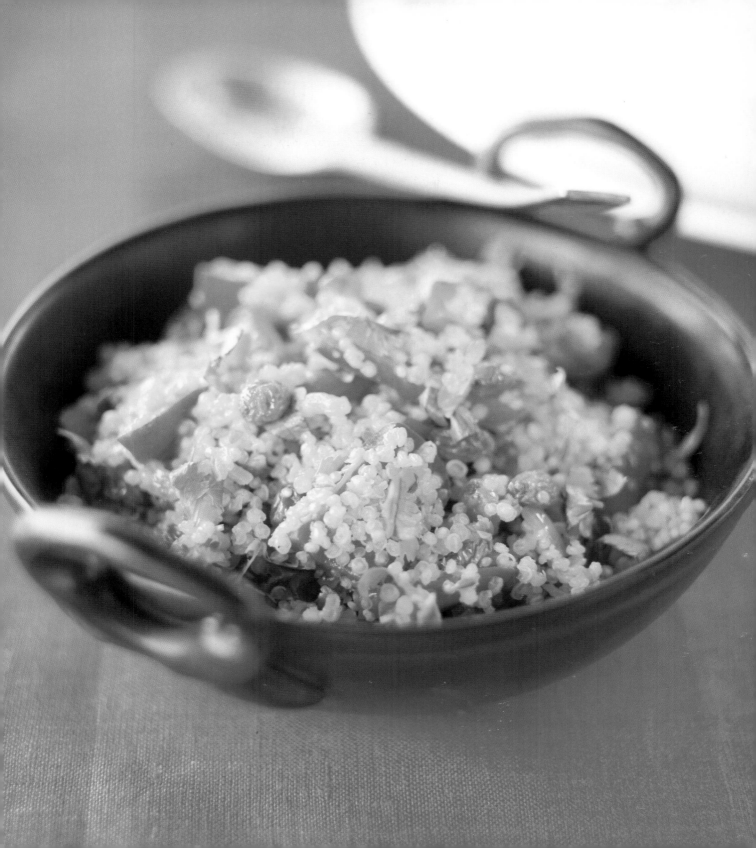

OAT-CRUSTED SALMON WITH SESAME SEEDS

MAKES 2 SERVINGS

The lightly toasted oat crust makes the fish lovely and crispy on the outside while adding extra flavour and nutrients. Serve this dish with steamed new potatoes and a salad of watercress and spinach.

300 g (10 oz) salmon fillet, skinned
2 tablespoon (30 ml) porridge oats
1 tablespoon (15 ml) sesame seeds
A little low-sodium salt and freshly ground black pepper
Lemon wedges to serve

▸ Cut the salmon in half.
▸ On a plate mix together the porridge oats, sesame seeds, low-sodium salt and black pepper.
▸ Dip each salmon portion in the oat mixture and press it all over so that the oats coat the fish evenly.
▸ Brush a non-stick frying pan or griddle with a little olive oil, allow it to heat up and then add the salmon. Cook over a moderate heat for 3 minutes on each side, covering with a lid. The salmon should be light brown and crispy on the outside. Serve with the lemon wedges.

HEALTH STATISTICS
Salmon is a concentrated source of omega-3 fatty acids, which help reduce the risk of heart attacks and stroke, as well as benefiting the skin, reducing the appearance of wrinkles and also helping to control blood pressure. Oats provide soluble fibre, which helps lower cholesterol levels and promote a healthy digestive tract.

NUTRITIONAL ANALYSIS (PER SERVING):

Calories 402 kcal	Carbohydrate 11 g
Protein 34 g	Total sugars* 0.1 g
Fat 25 g	Fibre 2.0 g
Saturates 3.9 g	Salt 0.2 g

* total sugars includes sugars found naturally in foods

VEGETABLE RISOTTO WITH CASHEW NUTS

MAKES 2 SERVINGS

A risotto is a great base for all sorts of vegetables. You can vary the vegetables according to what you have available and also add beans, different nuts and seeds.

2 tablespoons (30 ml) olive oil
1 small onion, chopped
1 small red pepper, chopped
1 garlic clove, crushed
1 bay leaf
150 g (5 oz) Arborio (risotto) rice
500 ml hot vegetable stock
85 g (3 oz) green beans, cut into 2-cm (3/4-in) lengths)
125 g (4 oz) frozen peas
2 tomatoes, deseeded and chopped
A handful of baby spinach leaves
Freshly ground black pepper.
60 g (2 oz) cashew nuts, lightly toasted

▸ Heat the olive oil in a large, heavy based pan and cook the onion with the red pepper, bay leaves and garlic over a moderate heat, stirring frequently.
▸ Stir in the rice and cook for 1–2 minutes, stirring constantly until the grains are coated with oil and translucent.
▸ Add half the hot vegetable stock and bring to the boil. Reduce the heat and simmer gently until the liquid is absorbed. Add the remaining stock, a ladleful at a time, stirring and continue to simmer until the rice is almost tender. Add the green beans, peas and tomatoes and continue cooking for a further 5 minutes. As a guide, the total cooking time should be around 25 minutes. Perfect risotto should be thick and creamy but not solid, and the rice should be soft but still have a little bite.
▸ Add the spinach leaves to the hot risotto. Stir until the leaves have wilted. Remove the pan from the heat.
▸ Season to taste with freshly ground black pepper then scatter over the cashew nuts. Serve on warmed plates.

HEALTH STATISTICS
Arborio rice has a lower glycaemic index than ordinary white rice so gives a steady release of energy and keeps you feeling nicely full for longer. This risotto provides lots of immunity-enhancing vitamin C from the red pepper, peas and spinach, as well as iron, beta-carotene and folic acid. The cashews supply heart-healthy monounsaturated oils, vitamin E and extra iron.

NUTRITIONAL ANALYSIS (PER SERVING):

Calories 498 kcal	Carbohydrate 60 g
Protein 16 g	Total sugars* 14 g
Fat 23 g	Fibre 8.8 g
Saturates 4.4 g	Salt 0.1 g

* total sugars includes sugars found naturally in foods

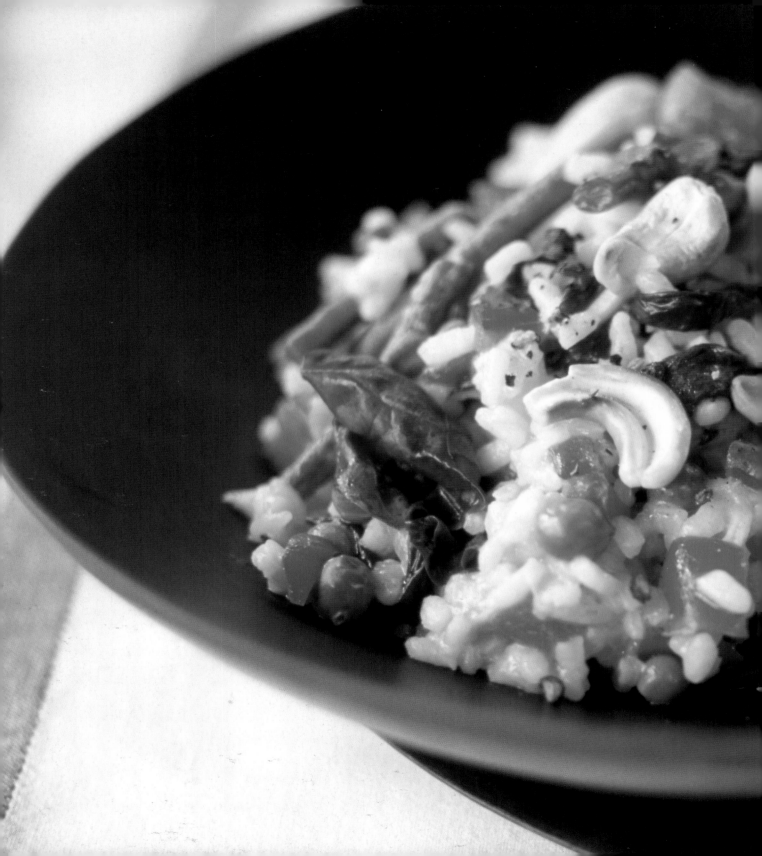

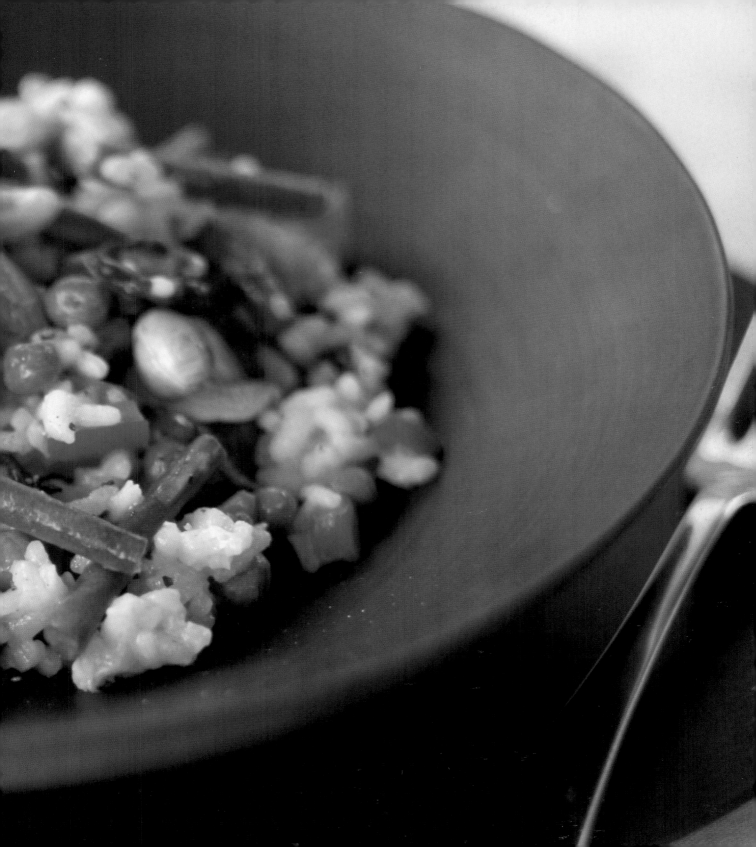

CHAPTER 7
SALADS

MANGO, LAMB'S LETTUCE AND TOMATO SALAD WITH PUMPKIN SEEDS

MAKES 2 SERVINGS

This may sound like an unlikely combination but the sweetness of the mango complements the slightly sweet-tasting tomatoes and lamb's lettuce beautifully. Substitute peaches (fresh or tinned) or apricots for the mango, if you prefer.

2 tablespoons (30 ml) pumpkin seeds
1 small ripe mango
1 bag (85 g/3 oz) of ready-washed lamb's lettuce
12 cherry tomatoes, halved
1 small red onion, sliced thinly

DRESSING:
1 tablespoon (15 ml) extra virgin olive oil
1 teaspoon (5 ml) walnut oil
2 teaspoons (10 ml) lemon juice

▸ Lightly toast the pumpkin seeds under a hot grill for about 5 minutes until they start to turn slightly brown and emit a wonderful nutty aroma. Allow to cool.
▸ Slice through the mango either side of the stone. Peel, then cut the flesh into cubes.
▸ Place the lamb's lettuce in a salad bowl. Combine with the mango, tomatoes and onion.
▸ For the dressing: place the extra virgin olive oil, walnut oil and lemon juice in a bottle or screw-top jar and shake together thoroughly. Pour over the salad, then toss gently.
▸ Scatter the toasted pumpkin seeds over the salad and serve.

HEALTH STATISTICS
Lamb's lettuce is an excellent source of iron, beta-carotene, folic acid and quercetin, a powerful antioxidant that can protect against cancer. Pumpkin seeds are rich in omega-3 oils as well as zinc, vitamin E and magnesium – all heart-healthy nutrients. Toasting them, as in this recipe, brings out their flavour.

NUTRITIONAL ANALYSIS (PER SERVING):

Calories 294 kcal	Carbohydrate 21 g
Protein 6.2 g	Total sugars* 17 g
Fat 21 g	Fibre 4.9 g
Saturates 3.1 g	Salt 0.1 g

* total sugars includes sugars found naturally in foods

GRILLED COURGETTE SALAD WITH MINT AND PINE NUTS

MAKES 2 SERVINGS

This lovely salad makes a perfect lunch served with some wholegrain bread or a side dish of cooked wholegrain rice.

2 large courgettes
1 tablespoon (15 ml) olive oil
1 garlic clove, crushed
Squeeze of lemon juice
100 g ready-washed watercress
2 plum tomatoes, sliced
Freshly ground black pepper
A few sprigs of fresh mint
2 tablespoons (30 ml) pine nuts

▸ Pre-heat the grill.
▸ Slice the courgettes thinly on the diagonal. Place on a baking tray. Drizzle over the olive oil, scatter over the crushed garlic and turn so that the vegetables are lightly coated in the oil.
▸ Grill the vegetables for around 5 minutes, turning once or twice during this time so that they cook on both sides. Squeeze over a little lemon juice, then set aside to cool.
▸ Divide the watercress between 2 plates. Arrange the courgettes and tomato slices on top, add the black pepper and scatter over the mint leaves and pine nuts.

HEALTH STATISTICS

Courgettes are rich in potassium and provide useful amounts of vitamin C and folate. Grilling them minimises the loss of these vitamins. Watercress is a terrfic source of iron, folate, and glucosinolates, plant nutrients that help prevent cancer.

NUTRITIONAL ANALYSIS (PER SERVING):

Calories 193 kcal	Carbohydrate 4.6 g
Protein 5.9 g	Total sugars* 4.5 g
Fat 17 g	Fibre 2.6 g
Saturates 1.8 g	Salt 0.1 g

* total sugars includes sugars found naturally in foods

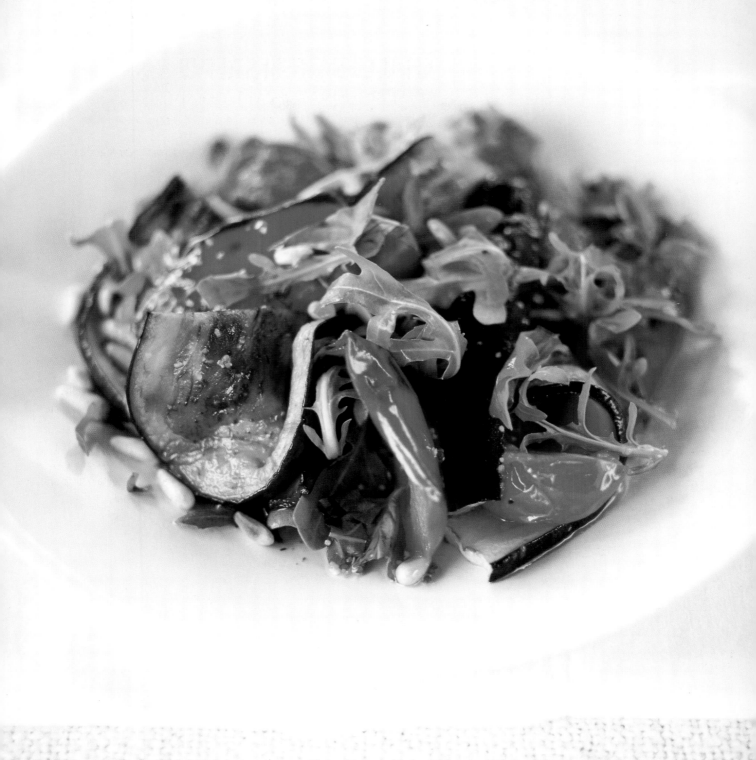

THAI CHICKEN SALAD

MAKES 2 SERVINGS

This wonderful medley of vegetables and chicken is good served with basmati rice.

400 ml coconut milk
Juice and rind of 2 limes
2 x 150 g (5 oz) skinless chicken breasts
½ romaine lettuce
½ bulb of fennel
15 cm (6 in) cucumber
1 large tomato
½ red or yellow pepper
2 spring onions
A handful of fresh mint, roughly torn
A small handful of peanuts

▸ Combine the coconut milk and the juice and rind of the limes in a saucepan. Add the chicken breasts. Bring to the boil, reduce the heat and poach the chicken gently for about 20 minutes. Remove them from the saucepan and leave to cool, then tear the chicken into large pieces.
▸ Cut the lettuce into wide ribbons. Halve, then thinly slice the fennel, discarding the tough inner 'core'. Slice the cucumber. Cut the tomatoes into quarters. Remove the seeds from the pepper and slice it thinly. Slice the spring onions.
▸ Combine the prepared salad vegetables with the chicken pieces in a large bowl. Add the mint leaves and scatter over the peanuts.

HEALTH STATISTICS
This dish provides good amounts of protein, B vitamins and fibre. Fennel adds useful amounts of beta-carotene, which helps promote healthy skin and protect against certain cancers, as well as potassium for regulating levels of fluid in the body. Coconut milk contains very few calories and has a low-fat content.

NUTRITIONAL ANALYSIS (PER SERVING):

Calories 268 kcal	Carbohydrate 17 g
Protein 34 g	Total sugars* 16 g
Fat 7.5 g	Fibre 3.1 g
Saturates 2.0 g	Salt 0.7 g

* total sugars includes sugars found naturally in foods

RICE AND BROAD BEAN SALAD WITH BALSAMIC DRESSING

MAKES 2 SERVINGS

Here's a salad you can throw together from store cupboard ingredients when you find you have nothing fresh in the fridge.

125 g (4 oz) wholegrain (brown) rice
300 g (10 oz) can broad beans, rinsed and drained
(or use cooked frozen beans)
125 g (4oz) canned sweetcorn, rinsed and drained
125 g (4 oz) baby plum tomatoes, halved
1 red pepper
1 tablespoon (15 ml) capers (optional)
2 tablespoons (30 ml) extra virgin olive oil
1 tablespoon (15 ml) balsamic vinegar
1/2 teaspoon (2.5 ml) wholegrain mustard

▸ Bring a large pan of water to the boil. Stir in the rice. Cover and simmer for the time recommended on the packet. Drain. Alternatively, cook the rice in twice its own volume of water until the water has been absorbed.
▸ Place the cooled rice in a large bowl with the broad beans and sweetcorn.
▸ Halve the baby plum tomatoes. Cut the red peppers into strips. Add to the rice mixture along with the capers and mix together.
▸ To make the dressing: put the oil, vinegar and mustard in a screw-top glass jar and shake well. Drizzle over the salad, toss well and serve.

HEALTH STATISTICS
Broad beans are rich in soluble fibre, which helps control blood cholesterol levels and is also responsible for their low glycaemic index. This means you'll have longer lasting energy and won't feel hungry between meals. They are also good sources of B vitamins and vitamin C.

NUTRITIONAL ANALYSIS (PER SERVING):

Calories 557 kcal	Carbohydrate 92 g
Protein 19 g	Total sugars* 16 g
Fat 15 g	Fibre 14 g
Saturates 2.4 g	Salt 0.5 g

* total sugars includes sugars found naturally in foods

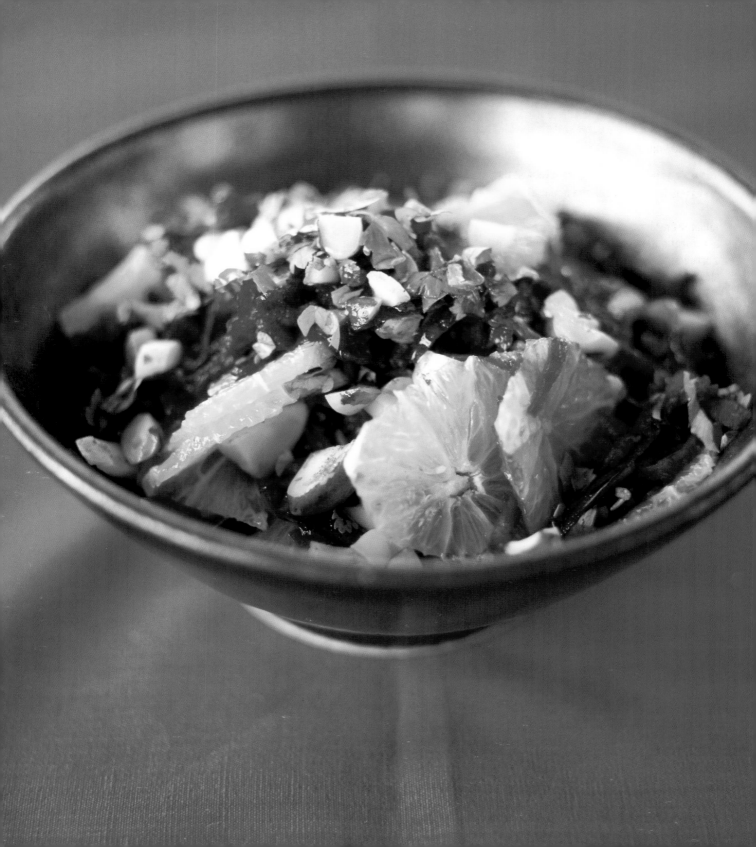

BEETROOT SALAD WITH CORIANDER AND BRAZIL NUTS

MAKES 2 SERVINGS

Not only does this amazing salad look stunning and taste delicious, it also saves you having to cook the beetroot!

About 10 Brazil nuts
2 raw beetroot
2 oranges
Small handful of fresh coriander, chopped
Juice of ½ lemon
1 teaspoon (5 ml) olive oil

▸ Lightly toast the Brazils on a baking tray under a pre heated grill. Shake the tin a couple of times to ensure even toasting. Take care not to burn them as they can turn quickly! Allow to cool, then chop roughly.

▸ Grate the beetroot (it is a good idea to wear rubber gloves for this to prevent staining your hands).

▸ Peel and thinly slice one of the oranges and mix with the beetroot and coriander in a medium-sized bowl.

▸ Squeeze the juice from the other orange and whisk with the lemon juice and olive oil. Pour over the beetroot mixture and mix gently. Scatter over the toasted Brazils and serve.

HEALTH STATISTICS

Raw beetroot is rich in iron, which promotes the production of red blood cells and improves the supply of oxygen to the cells. It is also a good source of folate, which helps to prevent heart attacks, and manganese, essential for brain function and bone strength. Its red colour comes from the pigment betanin, an antioxidant anthocyanin which can help fight cancer. It can also turn your urine pink – but don't worry, it is perfectly harmless!

NUTRITIONAL ANALYSIS (PER SERVING):

Calories 225 kcal	Carbohydrate 22 g
Protein 5.6 g	Total sugars* 21 g
Fat 14 g	Fibre 5.3 g
Saturates 2.9 g	Salt 0.1 g

* total sugars includes sugars found naturally in foods

TABBOULEH

MAKES 2 SERVINGS

This wonderfully fragrant summer salad is made with whole grains of cracked wheat, fresh herbs and lycopene-rich tomatoes.

85 g (3 oz) bulgar (cracked) wheat
A little low-sodium salt
Freshly ground black pepper
3 spring onions, finely chopped
1 tablespoon (15 ml) olive oil
Juice of ½ lemon
½ green pepper, deseeded and finely chopped
A handful of flat leaf parsley, chopped
A handful of mint leaves, chopped
3–4 small tomatoes, chopped

▸ Place the bulgar wheat in a bowl and add lukewarm water until just covered. Leave for 15 minutes, drain and then transfer back to the bowl. Season with the low-sodium salt and freshly ground black pepper.
▸ Add the spring onions, olive oil, lemon juice, green pepper, parsley, mint and tomatoes and combine all the ingredients together. Place in the fridge for at least 30 minutes to allow the flavours to infuse.

HEALTH STATISTICS
Bulgar wheat is rich in fibre, which promotes a healthy digestive system and helps lower your risk of bowel cancer. Like other wholegrains, it's also rich in iron (for healthy blood), zinc (for good immunity), selenium (for heart health) and vitamin E (for fighting free radicals). The tomatoes in this salad add cancer-protective lycopene and vitamin C, the green peppers provide extra vitamin C and the herbs are rich in iron and folate.

NUTRITIONAL ANALYSIS (PER SERVING):

Calories 226 kcal	Carbohydrate 37 g
Protein 5.4 g	Total sugars* 4.4 g
Fat 6.7 g	Fibre 1.8 g
Saturates 0.9 g	Salt 0.1 g

* total sugars includes sugars found naturally in foods

CHAR-GRILLED VEGETABLE SALAD WITH ROCKET AND PINE NUTS

MAKES 2 SERVINGS

I love making this salad in the summer when courgettes and tomatoes are plentiful. It's quick to make and can be varied infinitely according to which vegetables you have handy – try yellow or green peppers, quartered radicchio or fennel, or baby sweetcorn

1 courgette, sliced lengthways
1/2 aubergine, cut into thin slices
1 red pepper, deseeded and cut into wide strips
2 plum tomatoes
1 tablespoon (15 ml) extra virgin olive oil
1 bag (50 g/1³/₄ oz) rocket
2 tablespoons (30 ml) pine nuts
1 tablespoon (15 ml) basil leaves, torn

FOR THE DRESSING:
1 tablespoon (15 ml) extra virgin olive oil
1 teaspoon (5 ml) lemon juice
1/2 teaspoon (2.5 ml) wholegrain mustard
Freshly ground black pepper

▸ Pre-heat the grill.
▸ Place the prepared vegetables on a baking tray. Drizzle over the olive oil, and turn the vegetables gently so that they are lightly coated in the oil.
▸ Grill the vegetables, turning once, for around 2 minutes each side (or until slightly browned). Allow to cool.
▸ Place the rocket in a large salad bowl. Add the grilled vegetables and pine nuts.
▸ To make the dressing: place the olive oil, lemon juice, mustard and black pepper in a screw-top glass jar and shake well until mixed. Pour the dressing over the salad, toss well and scatter over the torn basil leaves.

HEALTH STATISTICS
This fibre-rich salad provides lots of vitamin C and beta-carotene, both powerful antioxidants that are protective against heart disease and many cancers. Grilling helps to conserve the vitamins as no water is used for cooking. Pine nuts, one of the anti-cellulite superfoods, are excellent sources of heart-healthy monounsaturated oils and vitamin E as well as iron and phosphorus.

NUTRITIONAL ANALYSIS (PER SERVING):

Calories 256 kcal	Carbohydrate 9.6 g
Protein 4.7 g	Total sugars* 9.2 g
Fat 2 g	Fibre 3.8 g
Saturates 2.6 g	Salt 0.1 g

* total sugars includes sugars found naturally in foods

AVOCADO AND GRAPEFRUIT SALAD WITH TOASTED PUMPKIN SEEDS

MAKES 2 SERVINGS

Avocados are one of my favourite salad ingredients, not only because they taste divine but also because they keep you feeling satisfied for a long time.

1 little gem lettuce, washed
1 ripe avocado
2 or 3 spring onions
½ grapefruit
A small handful of fresh coriander, roughly chopped
1 tablespoon (15 ml) extra virgin olive oil
1 tablespoon (15 ml) walnut oil
1 tablespoon (15 ml) lemon juice
Freshly ground black pepper
25 g (1 oz) pumpkin seeds

▸ Tear the lettuce into bite-sized pieces and place in a salad bowl.
▸ Cut the avocado into quarters, remove the stone and then peel carefully. Slice lengthways.
▸ Trim and coarsely chop the spring onions.
▸ Peel the grapefruit, removing all the white pith, and cut into segments.
▸ Combine the lettuce, avocado, spring onions, grapefruit and chopped coriander in the bowl.
▸ Shake the olive and walnut oils and lemon juice in a bottle or screw-top glass jar, then drizzle over the salad. Toss lightly, grind over the black pepper. Scatter over the pumpkin seeds and serve.

HEALTH STATISTICS

Avocados are excellent for your skin, helping to keep it smooth and prevent wrinkles. They are full of heart-healthy monounsaturated oils and vitamin E. The walnut oil in the dressing supplies extra omega-3 oils, which are also great for supple skin as well as preventing strokes and heart attacks. The grapefruit supplies lots of vitamin C and antioxidant bioflavanoids.

NUTRITIONAL ANALYSIS (PER SERVING):

Calories 330 kcal	Carbohydrate 7.1 g
Protein 5.5 g	Total sugars* 4.3 g
Fat 31 g	Fibre 4.4 g
Saturates 5.2 g	Salt 0.1 g

* total sugars includes sugars found naturally in foods

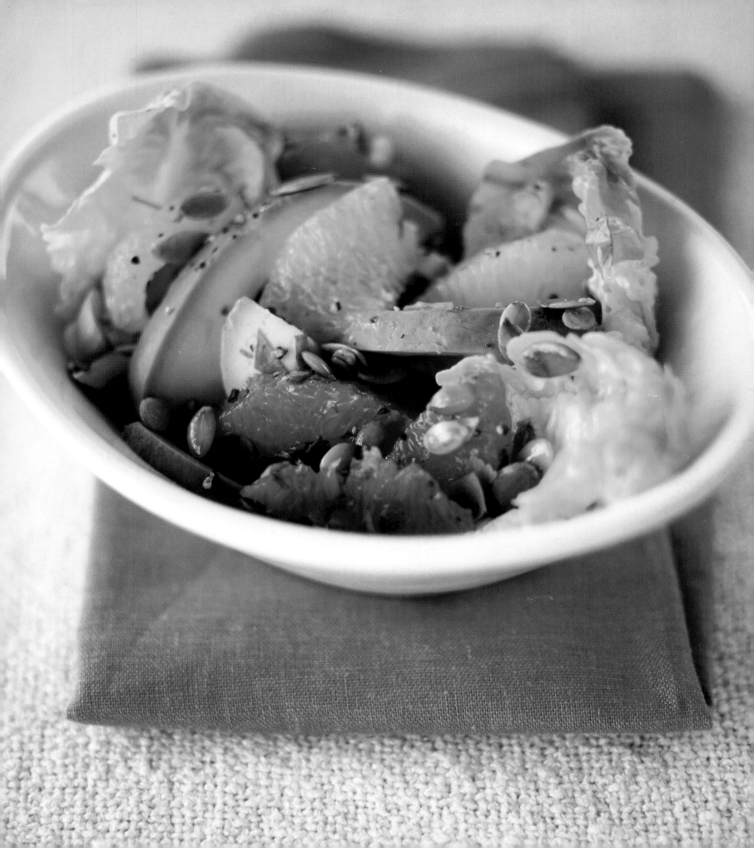

QUINOA AND ADUKI BEAN SALAD WITH HONEY DRESSING

MAKES 2 SERVINGS

Quinoa has a slightly nutty flavour, which complements the honey dressing and flaked almonds. Substitute other varieties of cooked or tinned beans for the aduki beans if you prefer.

85 g (3 oz) quinoa (available from
health food stores or larger supermarkets)
225 ml (8 fl oz) water or vegetable stock
200 g (7 oz) cooked aduki beans
(tinned or cooked dried beans)
4 spring onions, chopped
60 g (2 oz) cherry tomatoes, halved
25 g (1 oz) flaked toasted almonds

FOR THE DRESSING:
2 tablespoons (30 ml) extra virgin olive oil
2 teaspoons (10 ml) lemon juice
$1/2$ teaspoon (2.5 ml) clear honey
Low-sodium salt and freshly ground black
pepper

▸ Place the quinoa in a pan with the water or stock. Bring to the boil, then lower the heat, cover and simmer for about 20 minutes until the quinoa is tender. Remove from the heat, drain if necessary and transfer to a bowl.

▸ Add the aduki beans, spring onions, tomatoes and almonds and mix gently.

▸ To make the dressing: place the olive oil, lemon juice, honey, low-sodium salt and pepper in a screw-top glass jar and shake well until mixed. Pour the dressing over the salad and toss well until all the ingredients are coated in the dressing. Serve with a green salad.

HEALTH STATISTICS
The combination of quinoa and beans provides an excellent balance of protein and complex carbohydrates. It also results in a low glycaemic index, which will provide long lasting energy and stop you feeling hungry. The beans are rich in cholesterol-lowering fibre, iron and B vitamins, and the almonds provide added protein, calcium and vitamin E.

NUTRITIONAL ANALYSIS (PER SERVING)

Calories 447 kcal	Carbohydrate 50 g
Protein 18 g	Total sugars* 6.6 g
Fat 21 g	Fibre 7.0 g
Saturates 2.4 g	Salt 0.1 g

* total sugars includes sugars found naturally in foods

WARM BROCCOLI SALAD WITH WALNUT OIL

MAKES 2 SERVINGS

This salad is equally lovely in the winter or summer. Serve with new potatoes, grilled white fish or a simple mixed bean salad.

225 g (8 oz) small broccoli florets
1 small butterhead lettuce
1 tablespoon (15 ml) walnut oil
1 teaspoon (5 ml) lemon juice
1 garlic clove, crushed
Freshly ground black pepper

▸ Steam the broccoli for 3–5 minutes, until just tender but still crunchy. Drain, then place in a bowl.
▸ Tear the lettuce roughly and add to the broccoli. Combine.
▸ To make the dressing: shake the walnut oil, lemon juice and garlic in a bottle or screw-top glass jar, then drizzle over the salad. Toss lightly, grind over plenty of black pepper and serve.

HEALTH STATISTICS
This salad is packed with sulphoraphane, a powerful anti-cancer nutrient, which gives you significant protection from cancers of the lungs, breast, stomach, colon and rectum. There are also high levels of vitamin C and beta-carotene, which boost your immune system as well as protecting against heart disease. Steaming broccoli results in minimal losses of vitamin C and folate but make sure you eat it as soon as possible after cooking as losses increase once exposed to air.

NUTRITIONAL ANALYSIS (PER SERVING):

Calories 96 kcal	Carbohydrate 2.9 g
Protein 5.6 g	Total sugars* 2.4 g
Fat 7.0 g	Fibre 3.8 g
Saturates 0.8 g	Salt 0.1 g

* total sugars includes sugars found naturally in foods

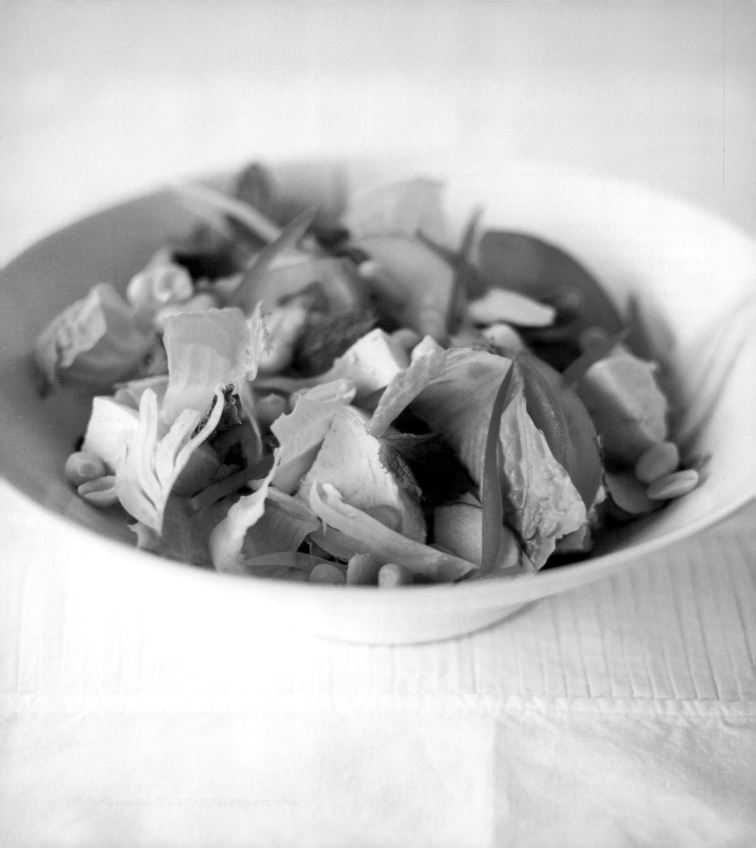

SPINACH AND TOFU SALAD WITH CASHEW NUTS

MAKE 2 SERVINGS

This super-quick salad makes a perfect lunch served with a little coarse-grain bread.

85 g (3 oz) ready-washed baby spinach leaves
1 small red onion, peeled and thinly sliced
1 orange, peeled and thinly sliced
1 tablespoon (15 ml) extra virgin olive oil
1 teaspoon (5 ml) lemon juice
1 teaspoon (5 ml) wholegrain mustard
125 g (4 oz) smoked tofu, diced
Freshly ground black pepper
60 g (2 oz) cashew nuts

▸ Place the spinach leaves in a large salad bowl. Add the onion and orange slices.
▸ Place the extra virgin olive oil, lemon juice and mustard in a bottle or screw-top jar and shake together thoroughly. Pour over the salad leaves, then toss so that every leaf is well coated with the dressing.
▸ Arrange the tofu on top of the salad and grind over some black pepper. Lightly crush the cashew nuts and scatter over the salad.

HEALTH STATISTICS
Spinach is rich in beta-carotene, which helps to keep your skin healthy and also prevent certain cancers. It also contains vitamin C (for keeping blood vessels healthy), folate (which helps prevent heart attacks) and iron (for healthy blood cells). Tofu is a great low-fat source of protein and calcium. The cashews provide extra protein as well as iron, zinc and vitamin E.

NUTRITIONAL ANALYSIS (PER SERVING):

Calories 318 kcal	Carbohydrate 16 g
Protein 13 g	Total sugars* 11 g
Fat 23 g	Fibre 3.6 g
Saturates 4.0 g	Salt 0.1 g

* total sugars includes sugars found naturally in foods

NEW POTATO AND CHICKEN SALAD

MAKES 2 SERVINGS

This quick salad makes a perfect mid-week supper.

2 tablespoons (30 ml) red wine vinegar
5 tablespoons (75 ml) water
2 teaspoons (10 ml) clear honey
2 tablespoons (30 ml) olive oil
A little low-sodium salt and freshly ground black pepper
2 boneless chicken breasts, skinned and cut into strips
225 g (8 oz) new potatoes
125 g cherry tomatoes
¹/₂ cucumber, diced
50 g bag rocket leaves

▸ Combine the vinegar, water, honey, 1 tablespoon of the oil, low-sodium salt and pepper in a bowl and add the chicken. Turn gently, then leave to marinate.
▸ Scrub the new potatoes and halve any large ones. Steam or boil for 10 minutes or until tender, then drain and allow to cool slightly. Mix with the tomatoes, cucumber and rocket.
▸ Heat the remaining oil in a large frying pan, remove the chicken from the marinade and stir fry for 8–10 minutes or until cooked through and lightly browned. Stir into the salad. Serve while still warm.

HEALTH STATISTICS
Chicken is a rich source of protein as well as B vitamins, which help release energy from carbohydrate foods. This salad also supplies plenty of vitamin C (from the tomatoes and rocket), beta-carotene, iron and folate.

NUTRITIONAL ANALYSIS (PER SERVING):

Calories 362 kcal	Carbohydrate 26 g
Protein 33 g	Total sugars* 9.6 g
Fat 15 g	Fibre 2.8 g
Saturates 2.7 g	Salt 0.2 g

* total sugars includes sugars found naturally in foods

LAMB'S LETTUCE, SPINACH AND GREEN BEAN SALAD WITH TARRAGON DRESSING

MAKES 2 SERVINGS

This elegant salad can either be served as a starter when entertaining or as a light lunch dish with a jacket potato and hummus.

85 g (3 oz) green beans
60 g (2 oz) lamb's lettuce
60 g (2 oz) baby spinach leaves
1 shallot, sliced thinly

FOR THE DRESSING:
2 tablespoons (30 ml) olive oil
1 tablespoon (15 ml) chopped tarragon
2 teaspoons (10 ml) cider vinegar
1/2 teaspoon (2.5 ml) clear honey

▸ Trim the green beans. Steam for 3–4 minutes until cooked al dente. Drain and refresh under cold running water.
▸ Place the beans in a bowl together with the salad leaves and shallot.
▸ Put the olive oil, tarragon, vinegar and honey in a screw-top glass jar, shake well, then pour the dressing over the salad.
▸ Toss lightly and serve.

HEALTH STATISTICS
Brimming with iron, folate and potassium, this salad also provides plenty of beta-carotene, which the body converts to vitamin A and bolsters the immune system. Spinach helps to protect against breast, cervical and lung cancers as well as helping fight heart disease. Its vitamin C content helps to strengthen blood vessels and connective tissue, thus helping improve the appearance of cellulite.

NUTRITIONAL ANALYSIS (PER SERVING):

Calories 131 kcal	Carbohydrate 3.8 g
Protein 2.7 g	Total sugars* 3.4 g
Fat 12 g	Fibre 2.3 g
Saturates 1.7 g	Salt 0.1 g

* total sugars includes sugars found naturally in foods

WARM LENTIL SALAD WITH BABY SPINACH AND WALNUTS

MAKES 2 SERVINGS

You can make this salad with dried or tinned lentils. I like it warm, but it's equally good when eaten cold.

400 g (14oz) tin brown lentils
(or 125 g (4 oz) dried lentils, soaked
and boiled for 30 minutes)
4 spring onions, finely chopped
125 g (4 oz) cherry tomatoes, halved
60 g (2 oz) walnut pieces
1 tablespoon (15 ml) mint leaves,
roughly chopped
Juice of ½ lime
3 tablespoons (45 ml) extra virgin olive oil
1 tablespoon (15 ml) red wine vinegar
A little low-sodium salt and freshly ground
black pepper
2 handfuls ready-washed baby spinach leaves,
approximately 125 g (4 oz)

▸ Put the lentils in a saucepan with 2 tablespoons of water and warm through for a few minutes. Drain and transfer to a bowl.
▸ Mix with the spring onions, tomatoes, walnuts and chopped mint.
▸ Place the lime juice, olive oil and red wine vinegar in a bottle or screw-top glass jar and shake together. Pour the dressing over the warm lentils.
▸ Toss lightly and season with low-sodium salt and pepper.
▸ Arrange the baby spinach leaves on a serving plate and pile the lentil salad on top.

HEALTH STATISTICS

Brown lentils are extremely rich in iron, which is absorbed particularly well when eaten with the tomatoes. The vitamin C in the tomatoes aids the uptake of iron. This recipes also provides plenty of protein, B vitamins and fibre and the spinach is a good source of folate and calcium.

NUTRITIONAL ANALYSIS (PER SERVING):

Calories 547 kcal	Carbohydrate 38 g
Protein 25 g	Total sugars* 5.0 g
Fat 34 g	Fibre 11 g
Saturates 3.6 g	Salt 0.3 g

* total sugars includes sugars found naturally in foods

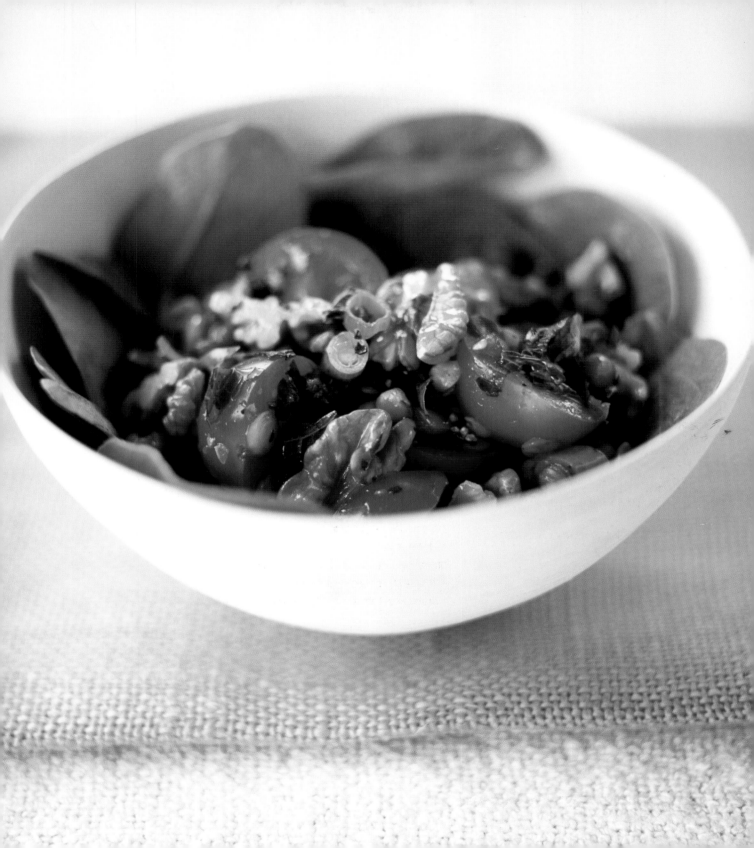

CHAPTER 8
VEGETABLES

ROASTED PEPPERS WITH TOMATOES, OLIVES AND ROCKET

MAKES 2 SERVINGS

1 red and 1 yellow pepper
2 tablespoons (30 ml) olive oil
2 tomatoes
1 garlic clove, crushed
12 pitted black olives
50 g (1 bag ready washed) rocket

▸ Heat the oven to 190°C/375°F/Gas Mark 5.
▸ Cut the peppers in quarters lengthways, remove the seeds then place them in a roasting tin. Quarter the tomatoes and add to the tin. Drizzle the oil over the vegetables and toss gently until they are well-coated in oil. Roast for 20 minutes until softened.
▸ Scatter the garlic and olives over the vegetables and return to the oven for a further 5 minutes.
▸ Take the vegetables out of the oven and divide between two plates then scatter over the rocket.
▸ Serve with a little low-fat natural yoghurt mixed with a little lemon juice.

HEALTH STATISTICS
One portion of this dish gives you your daily requirement for vitamin C. This vitamin is a terrific immunity booster as well as an established antioxidant that helps defend against free-radical damage and promotes healthy skin. It is found in abundance in peppers and tomatoes. The olives add extra vitamin E and heart-healthy monounsaturated oils.

NUTRITIONAL ANALYSIS (PER SERVING):

Calories 185 kcal	Carbohydrate 11 g
Protein 3.5 g	Total sugars* 11 g
Fat 14 g	Fibre 4.6 g
Saturates 2.1 g	Salt 1.4 g**

* total sugars includes sugars found naturally in foods
** this figure will be lower if you rinse the olives or use olives in olive oil rather than brine

ROASTED SQUASH WITH ROSEMARY

MAKES 2 SERVINGS

¹/₂ butternut squash
A few sprigs of fresh or dried rosemary
1 garlic clove, crushed
Freshly ground black pepper
2 tablespoons (30 ml) olive oil

▸ Pre-heat the oven to 200°C/400°F/Gas mark 6.
▸ Peel and deseed the butternut squash then cut into large wedges. Place them in a large roasting tin.
▸ Scatter over the rosemary, crushed garlic, and plenty of freshly ground black pepper. Drizzle over the olive oil, then turn the squash so it is coated in oil.
▸ Roast for 35–40 minutes until softened.
▸ Serve with baked potatoes, a leafy salad and a few walnuts or pine nuts for extra protein.

HEALTH STATISTICS

Butternut squash is packed with beta-carotene, a powerful antioxidant that helps protect against cancer and heart disease as well as protect your skin against UV light damage, wrinkling and premature aging. It is also one of the richest vegetable sources of heart-protective vitamin E.

NUTRITIONAL ANALYSIS (PER SERVING):

Calories 135 kcal	Carbohydrate 8.3 g
Protein 1.1 g	Total sugars* 4.5 g
Fat 11 g	Fibre 1.6 g
Saturates 1.6 g	Salt 0.1 g

* total sugars includes sugars found naturally in foods

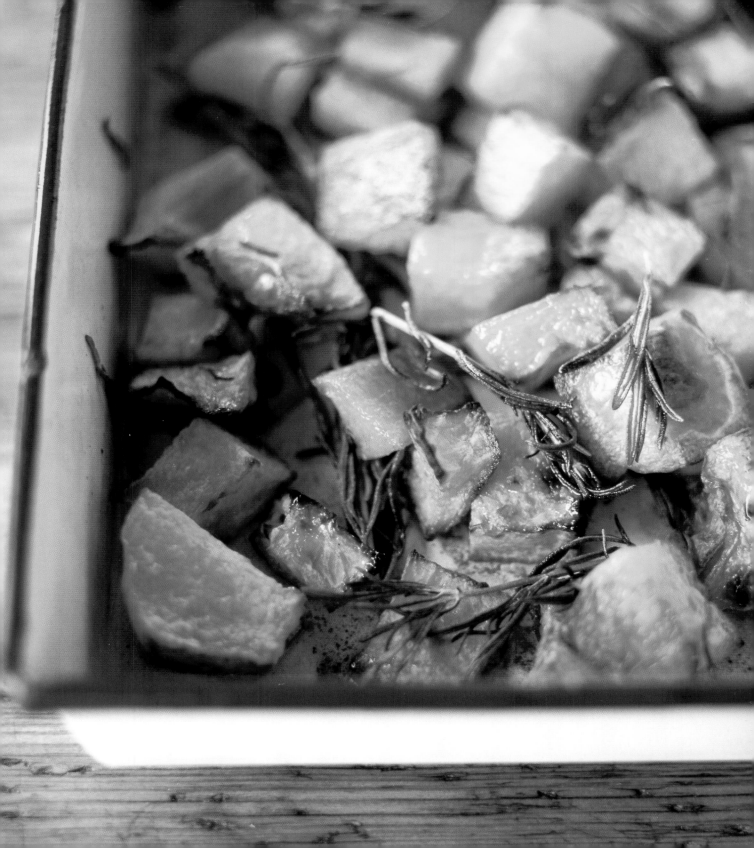

ROASTED VEGETABLES WITH MARINATED TOFU

MAKES 2 SERVINGS

1 small red onion, roughly sliced
$^1/_2$ red pepper, cut in to strips
$^1/_2$ yellow pepper, cut in to strips
$^1/_2$ orange pepper, cut in to strips
1 small courgette, trimmed and thickly sliced
$^1/_2$ aubergine, cut into 2-cm ($^3/_4$-in) cubes
2 garlic cloves, crushed
1–2 tablespoons (15–30 ml) extra virgin olive oil
85 g (3 oz) marinated tofu pieces
Freshly ground black pepper
A small handful of fresh basil, roughly torn

▸ Pre-heat the oven to 200°C/400°F/Gas Mark 6.
▸ Place the prepared vegetables in a large roasting tin and scatter over the crushed garlic. Pour over the olive oil and toss lightly, thoroughly coating the vegetables.
▸ Roast in the oven for about 25 minutes, turning them occasionally. Scatter the tofu pieces over and continue roasting for 5 minutes until the vegetables are slightly charred on the outside and tender in the middle.
▸ Remove from the oven and spoon onto a serving dish. Grind over the black pepper and sprinkle with the torn basil.

HEALTH STATISTICS
Peppers are one of the richest sources of vitamin C as well as many other phytonutrients that support the immune system and protect the body from free-radical damage. Roasting them in a small quantity of olive oil, as in this recipe, minimises any destruction of vitamins. The tofu provides good amounts of protein, important for cell repair and renewal, as well as bone-strengthening calcium.

NUTRITIONAL ANALYSIS (PER SERVING):

Calories 143 kcal	Carbohydrate 12 g
Protein 6.2 g	Total sugars* 11 g
Fat 8.1 g	Fibre 3.4 g
Saturates 1.2 g	Salt 0.1 g

* total sugars includes sugars found naturally in foods

WALNUT AND PECAN BURGERS

MAKES 8

These burgers are really easy to make if you have a food processor.
Not only are they super-nutritious, but they are perfect for vegetarian guests
at a barbecue. This recipe makes 8, so if you don't need them all, freeze the
remainder (for up to 3 months) for another meal.

60 g (2 oz) walnuts
125 g (4 oz) pecans
140 g (4½ oz) fresh wholemeal breadcrumbs
1 large red onion, finely chopped
1 garlic clove, crushed
1 teaspoon (5ml) dried rosemary
A little low-sodium salt and freshly ground black pepper
2 omega-3 rich eggs

▸ Pre-heat the oven to 190°C/375°F/Gas Mark 5.
▸ Place the nuts in a food processor and whizz until they are finely ground. Add the
breadcrumbs with the onions, garlic, rosemary, low-sodium salt and freshly ground
black pepper. Process the mixture for about 30 minutes until it is evenly combined.
Add the eggs and process until the mixture holds together firmly. If it is too wet, add
a few more breadcrumbs.
▸ Form the mixture into 8 flat burgers 1.5 cm (½ inch) thick.
▸ Place them on an oiled baking tray, then brush with olive oil . Bake in the oven for
25–30 minutes until they are crisp and brown.

HEALTH STATISTICS
Walnuts and pecans are a great source of heart-
healthy omega-3 oils, which are important for
regulating hormone levels, promoting healthy
joints and preventing clots forming in the
arteries. They also supply protein, iron, vitamin E
and zinc.

NUTRITIONAL ANALYSIS (PER BURGER):

Calories 230 kcal	Carbohydrate 11 g
Protein 6.3 g	Total sugars* 3.0 g
Fat 18 g	Fibre 2.3 g
Saturates 1.8 g	Salt 0.3 g

* total sugars includes sugars found naturally in foods

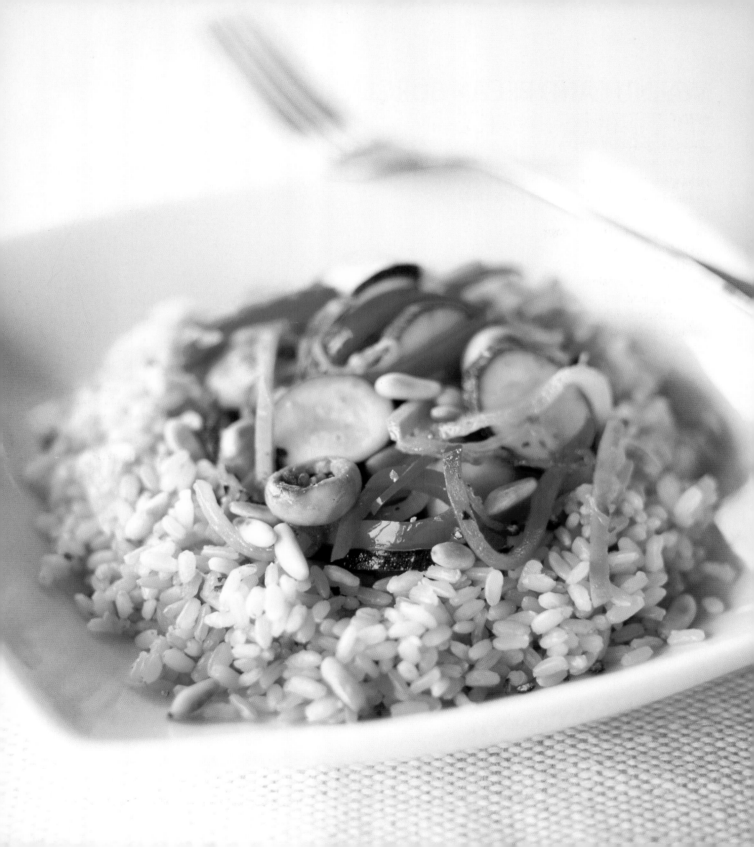

NEST OF STIR-FRIED VEGETABLES ON RICE

MAKES 2 SERVINGS

1 tablespoon (15 ml) olive oil
1 teaspoon (5 ml) sesame oil
1 small onion, sliced
1 teaspoon (5 ml) grated fresh ginger
1 garlic clove, crushed
½ red pepper, sliced
1 carrot, cut into thin batons
1 courgette, sliced
85 g (3oz) button mushrooms
2 tablespoons (30 ml) pine nuts
125 g (4 oz) brown or wild rice

▸ Heat the oils in a non-stick wok or large frying pan. Add the onion, ginger and garlic and stir-fry for 2 minutes.

▸ Add the peppers and carrots and stir-fry for a further 2–3 minutes.

▸ Add the remaining vegetables and continue stir-frying for a further 2 minutes. Stir in the pine nuts.

▸ Wash the rice. Add to a large pan of water and bring to the boil. Reduce the heat and simmer for 30–35 minutes until the grains are tender. Drain and fluff up the rice. Arrange a circular nest of rice on two plates. Fill each rice nest with the stir-fried vegetables and serve immediately.

HEALTH STATISTICS
Stir-frying helps preserve the vitamins in the vegetables because they are cooked only briefly at a high temperature and no vitamins are lost in cooking liquid. This recipe is a good source of vitamin C, fibre and vitamin E. Pine nuts and olive and sesame oils are excellent sources of unsaturated oils, which benefit the skin, keeping it smooth and supple.

NUTRITIONAL ANALYSIS (PER SERVING):

Calories 441 kcal	Carbohydrate 61 g
Protein 9.0 g	Total sugars* 9.4 g
Fat 20 g	Fibre 4.4 g
Saturates 2.3 g	Salt 0.1 g

* total sugars includes sugars found naturally in foods

GRIDDLED TOFU WITH STIR FRIED GREENS AND SESAME SEEDS

MAKES 2 SERVINGS

250 g (8 oz) firm tofu
1 garlic clove, crushed
1 teaspoon (5 ml) grated fresh ginger
1 tablespoon (15 ml) low-sodium soy sauce
2 tablespoons (30 ml) water
1 tablespoon (15 ml) sesame oil
½ onion, thinly sliced
1 garlic clove, crushed
85 g (3 oz) shitake or chestnut mushrooms, sliced
125 g (4 oz) spring cabbage, shredded
60 g (2 oz) bean sprouts
2 teaspoons (10 ml) sesame seeds

HEALTH STATISTICS
Tofu is an excellent low-fat, vegetarian source of protein and calcium. It also contains phytoestrogens, which may reduce certain menopausal symptoms, such as hot flushes. Spring greens are rich in folate, iron, beta-carotene and vitamin C, while the sesame seeds provide useful amounts of vitamin E and zinc.

NUTRITIONAL ANALYSIS (PER SERVING):

Calories 222 kcal	Carbohydrate 10 g
Protein 15 g	Total sugars* 7.0 g
Fat 14 g	Fibre 3.6 g
Saturates 1.9 g	Salt 0.1 g

* total sugars includes sugars found naturally in foods

▸ Cut the block of tofu in half and then into triangles about 5 mm thick. Put them into a shallow dish. Mix together the garlic, ginger, soy sauce and water and pour over the tofu, making sure it covers each piece.

▸ Heat the oil in a wok, add the onion and garlic and stir-fry for 1 minute, then add the other prepared vegetables and fry for 3–5 minutes, stirring frequently, until the cabbage is tender but still crisp.

▸ Brush the griddle pan (or wok, if you don't have a griddle pan) with a little oil and heat. Drain the tofu and place each piece carefully on the pan. You may need to do this in 2 or 3 batches. Cook for 2 minutes on each side until the tofu is seared with brown stripes. Turn the pieces over and cook the other side.

▸ Drizzle any remaining marinade over the stir-fried vegetables, stir and divide onto two plates. Top with the tofu and scatter the sesame seeds over the dish.

GRILLED COURGETTES WITH MINT AND LEMON

MAKES 2 SERVINGS

This simple dish is excellent served as a starter or, accompanied with a big salad and grilled fish or a lentil dish.

2 medium courgettes
2 tablespoons (30 ml) olive oil
1 tablespoon (15 ml) lemon juice
Small handful fresh mint leaves, roughly torn

▸ Pre-heat the grill.
▸ Slice the courgettes lengthways. Place them on a baking tray. Brush with a little olive oil and grill for 2–3 minutes on each side. Place them in a shallow dish.
▸ Put the olive oil, lemon juice and mint in a bowl, mix, then pour over the courgettes. Cover and marinate for at least 1 hour.

HEALTH STATISTICS
Courgettes are very low in calories – most of the calories in this recipe come from the heart-healthy olive oil. Courgettes are good sources of vitamin C, which is retained in this recipe as the courgettes are eaten raw. They also provide useful amounts of several minerals, including potassium, magnesium and iron.

NUTRITIONAL ANALYSIS (PER SERVING):

Calories 117 kcal	Carbohydrate 1.8 g
Protein 1.8 g	Total sugars* 1.7 g
Fat 11 g	Fibre 0.9 g
Saturates 1.7 g	Salt 0.1 g

* total sugars includes sugars found naturally in foods

TOFU AND MUSHROOM KEBABS

MAKES 2 SERVINGS

These kebabs are perfect for al fresco dining and barbecues.

FOR THE MARINADE:
2 tablespoons (30 ml) olive oil
1 tablespoon (15 ml) low sodium soy sauce
½ teaspoon (2.5 ml) grated fresh root ginger
1 teaspoon (5 ml) clear honey
1 garlic clove, crushed
1–2 tablespoons (15–30 ml) water

125 g (4 oz) firm tofu (plain or smoked), cut into chunks
1 red or yellow pepper, de-seeded and cut into 2.5-cm (1-in) pieces
½ aubergine, cut into bite-sized pieces
16 button mushrooms

▸ To make the marinade, mix together the olive oil, soy sauce, ginger, honey, garlic and water.
▸ Place the tofu, peppers, aubergine and mushrooms in a shallow dish, pour over the marinade, turn gently, making sure they are thoroughly coated. Leave covered for at about 30 minutes (or longer), turning occasionally.
▸ Preheat the grill and line the grill rack with foil.
▸ Thread the tofu and vegetables onto 4 wooden skewers . Brush with the remaining marinade and place under the hot grill for about 10 minutes, turning frequently and brushing with marinade until slightly browned.
▸ Serve with cooked wholegrain rice and a green salad .

HEALTH STATISTICS
Marinating vegetables in olive oil before grilling is healthy because the oil is mostly the healthy monounsaturated kind, which features heavily in the Mediterranean diet. It helps to lower blood cholesterol levels, in particular the 'bad' LDL cholesterol, thus protecting against heart disease. The tofu in this recipe provides useful protein and calcium while the mushrooms provide B vitamins.

NUTRITIONAL ANALYSIS (PER SERVING):

Calories 211 kcal	Carbohydrate 14 g
Protein 7.4 g	Total sugars* 12 g
Fat 14 g	Fibre 2.7 g
Saturates 2.1 g	Salt 0.1 g

* total sugars includes sugars found naturally in foods

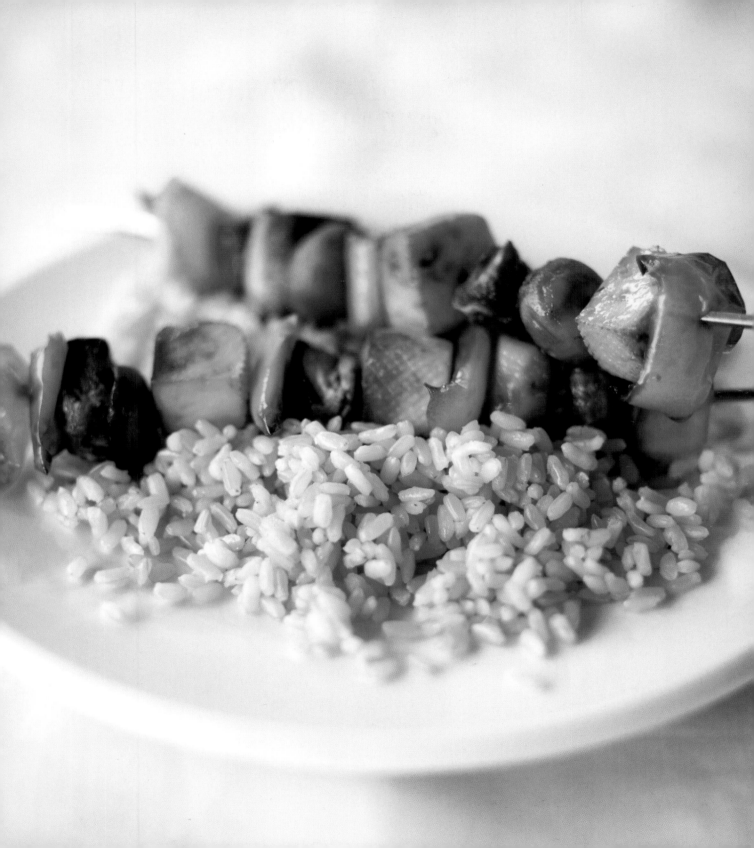

AUBERGINES WITH TOMATOES AND MUSHROOMS

MAKES 2 SERVINGS

1 large aubergine
4 tomatoes
1 onion
4 large mushrooms
1 garlic clove, crushed
A few sprigs of thyme
A little low-sodium salt and freshly ground black pepper
2 tablespoons (30 ml) olive oil

▸ Heat the oven to 190°C/375°F/Gas Mark 5.
▸ Cut the aubergine and tomatoes into ½ -cm (¼-in) slices. Peel and thinly slice the onion. Wipe and slice the mushrooms. Arrange alternating slices of aubergine, tomato, onion and mushrooms in an ovenproof baking dish. Scatter over the garlic, and thyme. Season with low-sodium salt and pepper and drizzle over the olive oil. Toss gently until the vegetables are well-coated in oil. Bake in the oven for 25 minutes or until the vegetables are softened.
▸ Serve with grilled fish or a little goat's cheese and steamed new potatoes.

HEALTH STATISTICS
This dish provides healthy monounsaturated oil, which benefits your heart and circulatory system, as well as good amounts of fibre, potassium and vitamin C. Aubergines contain a type of antioxidant called nausin (which gives the skin its glossy purple colour). It blocks the formation of free radicals, which helps protect against damage to cell membranes and reduces the risk of atherosclerosis.

NUTRITIONAL ANALYSIS (PER SERVING):

Calories 145 kcal	Carbohydrate 8.3 g
Protein 2.4 g	Total sugars* 6.3 g
Fat 12 g	Fibre 3.4 g
Saturates 1.7 g	Salt 0.1 g

* total sugars includes sugars found naturally in foods

VEGETABLE CURRY WITH BLACK-EYE BEANS AND ALMONDS

MAKES 2 SERVINGS

This lightly spiced curry is perfect on a cold evening. Serve with brown rice or wholewheat chapattis. Make a larger quantity and keep the remaining portions in the fridge for up to 3 days or freeze for up to 3 months.

1 carrot, sliced

1 medium potato, peeled and cut into cubes

½ butternut squash, peeled and cut into cubes

125 g (4 oz) broccoli florets

60 g (2 oz) frozen peas

2 tablespoons (30 ml) olive oil

1 onion, sliced

½ teaspoon (2.5 ml) of each: cumin, coriander and turmeric

1 garlic clove, crushed

1 teaspoon (5 ml) grated fresh ginger

200 g (7 oz) tinned chopped tomatoes

1 tablespoon (15 ml) desiccated coconut

200 ml (7 fl oz) plain yoghurt

25 g (1oz) ground almonds

225g (8oz) tinned black-eye beans, rinsed and drained

A small handful fresh coriander leaves, chopped

A little low-sodium salt and freshly ground black pepper

▸ Boil or steam the carrot, potato, butternut squash and broccoli for 5 minutes. Add the peas and cook for a further 3 minutes. Drain the vegetables and put aside.

▸ Heat the oil in a large pan and add the onion. Cook gently for 5 minutes until softened. Add the spices, garlic and ginger and cook for a further minute, then add the tomatoes. Bring to the boil and cook for 2–3 minutes.

▸ In a separate bowl, mix together the coconut, yoghurt and almonds.

▸ Add the cooked vegetables and black-eye beans to the tomato mixture and simmer for a few minutes.

▸ Finally, stir in the yoghurt mixture . Turn off the heat, taking care not to boil, otherwise the yoghurt may curdle. Stir in the coriander and season with low-sodium salt and freshly ground black pepper.

HEALTH STATISTICS

This dish is brimming with vitamins, minerals and antioxidant nutrients. The vegetables supply vitamins A and C as well as fibre, all of which delivers a powerful cancer-fighting punch. The beans provide protein, complex carbohydrates and cholesterol-lowering fibre, while the yoghurt gives added calcium for strong bones.

NUTRITIONAL ANALYSIS (PER SERVING):

Calories 551 kcal	Carbohydrate 65 g
Protein 26 g	Total sugars* 22 g
Fat 23 g	Fibre 13 g
Saturates 4.6 g	Salt 0.3 g

* total sugars includes sugars found naturally in foods

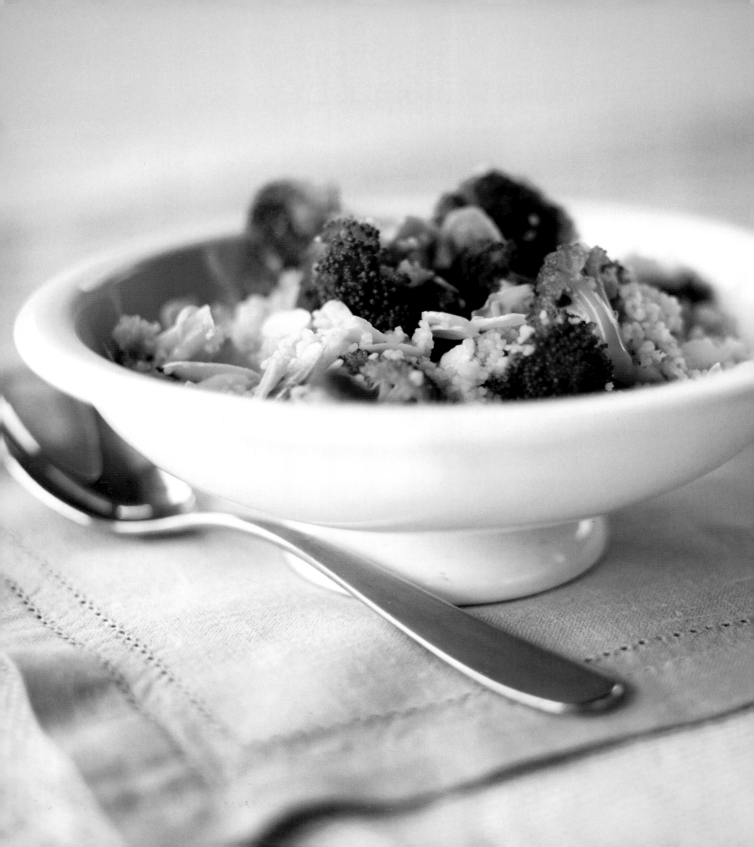

BROCCOLI WITH CINNAMON COUSCOUS AND ALMONDS

MAKES 2 SERVINGS

Couscous is really easy to prepare. It's also filling but without too many calories. In this recipe, it is flavoured with cinnamon, which goes perfectly with the broccoli and almonds.

125g (4 oz) couscous
175g (6 oz) small broccoli florets
Large pinch ground cinnamon
1 tablespoon (15 ml) olive oil
25g (1 oz) toasted flaked almonds
A little low-sodium salt and freshly ground black pepper

▸ Put the couscous in a large bowl and pour over 200 ml boiling water. Cover and leave for 10 minutes.
▸ Meanwhile, trim the broccoli then steam for 3–4 minutes until tender-crisp. Drain.
▸ Stir the cinnamon into the couscous and fluff up with a fork. Add the broccoli, olive oil, toasted almonds and seasoning. Mix well and serve warm.

HEALTH STATISTICS
Broccoli is an excellent source of sulphoraphane, a powerful anti-cancer nutrient, which protects against cancers of the lungs, breast, stomach, colon and rectum. There are also high levels of vitamin C and beta-carotene, which boost your immune system as well as protect against heart disease. Almonds add protein and calcium to this dish.

NUTRITIONAL ANALYSIS (PER SERVING):

Calories 298 kcal	Carbohydrate 35 g
Protein 10 g	Total sugars* 1.6 g
Fat 14 g	Fibre 3.2 g
Saturates 1.6 g	Salt 0.1 g

* total sugars includes sugars found naturally in foods

CHAPTER 9
SOUP

TOMATO AND CHICKPEA MINESTRONE SOUP

MAKES 2 SERVINGS

Try this interesting twist on standard minestrone soup. You can substitute other varieties of tinned beans, such as cannelloni or borlotti beans, if you wish.

500 ml (16 fl oz) vegetable stock
1 small red onion, chopped
1–2 garlic cloves, crushed
400 g (14 oz) tinned chopped tomatoes
200g (7 oz) tinned chickpeas
1 small courgette, trimmed and finely sliced
60 g (2 oz) fine green beans
60g (2 oz) small wholewheat pasta shapes
Small handful basil leaves, torn
1 tablespoon (15 ml) omega-3 rich oil or olive oil

▸ Pour the vegetable stock into a large saucepan. Bring to the boil and add the onion, garlic, tomatoes, chickpeas, courgettes and green beans. Lower the heat, cover and simmer for 10 minutes until the vegetables are tender.
▸ Add the pasta and continue cooking for a further 3–5 minutes or according to the cooking times on the packet. Stir in the torn basil leaves.
▸ Serve the soup hot in individual bowls. Drizzle with the oil.

HEALTH STATISTICS
This soup is rich in fibre, potassium, vitamin C and fibre. The chickpeas supply protein, B vitamins and complex carbohydrates with a low glycaemic index. The tomatoes are a good source of beta-carotene, vitamins C and E, as well as lycopene, which helps reduce the risk of heart disease and cancer.

NUTRITIONAL ANALYSIS (PER SERVING):

Calories 328 kcal	Carbohydrate 49 g
Protein 15 g	Total sugars* 9.9 g
Fat 9.5 g	Fibre 9.5 g
Saturates 1.3 g	Salt 0.8 g

* total sugars includes sugars found naturally in foods

EASY CARROT SOUP

MAKES 2 SERVINGS

One of the easiest vegetable soups to make and packed with vital nutrients, this is a firm winter favourite with my family.

1 onion, finely chopped
1 garlic clove, crushed
4 carrots, sliced
1 medium potato, peeled and chopped
500 ml (16 fl oz) vegetable stock
Freshly ground black pepper
1 tablespoon (15 ml) omega-3 rich oil or olive oil
1 tablespoon (15 ml) fresh parsley, finely chopped

▸ Place the onion, garlic, carrots and potato in a large saucepan. Add the stock and bring to the boil, then reduce the heat and simmer for 15 minutes until the vegetables are tender. Allow the soup to cool slightly for a couple of minutes. Season with the freshly ground black pepper and add the oil.
▸ Liquidise the soup using a hand blender or conventional blender, then stir in the fresh parsley.

HEALTH STATISTICS
This soup is an excellent source of beta-carotene, a powerful antioxidant that helps combat free radicals which cause cancer. It is also good for strengthening the skin and boosting its natural defences against the damaging effects of ultra-violet light.

NUTRITIONAL ANALYSIS (PER SERVING):

Calories 198 kcal	Carbohydrate 34 g
Protein 3.7 g	Total sugars* 17 g
Fat 6.3 g	Fibre 6.0 g
Saturates 1.0 g	Salt 0.1 g

* total sugars includes sugars found naturally in foods

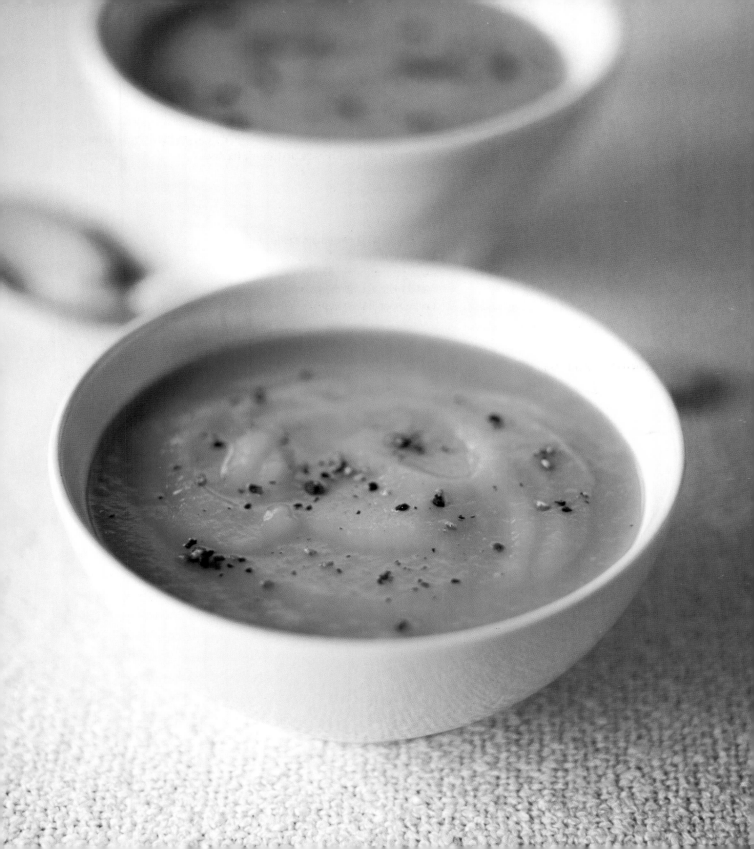

SPICY LENTIL SOUP

MAKES 2 SERVINGS

This soup is hearty and filling. You can add extra vegetables, such as carrots and mushrooms, to boost the nutritional and fibre value further.

1–2 teaspoons (5–10 ml) curry paste
1 onion, chopped
1 garlic clove, crushed
2-cm (³/₄-in) piece root ginger, peeled and finely chopped
125g (4oz) red lentils
500 ml (16 fl oz) vegetable stock
Grated zest and juice of 1 lime
A little low-sodium salt and freshly ground black pepper
Chopped fresh mint to garnish

▸ Place the curry paste, onion, garlic and ginger in a large pan and cook gently for three minutes.
▸ Add the lentils and vegetable stock and bring to the boil. Reduce the heat and simmer for 20 minutes. Add the lime zest and juice, bring back to the boil and simmer for a further 10 minutes until the lentils are soft. Season to taste with low-sodium salt and pepper.
▸ Ladle into bowls and garnish with the mint leaves.

HEALTH STATISTICS
This soup provides a near-perfect balance of nutrients. Lentils are low in fat and high in protein as well as an excellent source of complex carbohydrates and fibre. They also supply iron, B vitamins, zinc, and selenium, which makes them powerful nutrient powerhouses.

NUTRITIONAL ANALYSIS (PER SERVING):

Calories 232 kcal	Carbohydrate 41 g
Protein 16 g	Total sugars* 5.8 g
Fat 1.5 g	Fibre 4.1 g
Saturates 0.1 g	Salt 0.2 g

* total sugars includes sugars found naturally in foods

BUTTERNUT SQUASH AND CARROT SOUP

MAKES 2 SERVINGS

This soup makes a perfect lunch when it's cold outside. It's really warming and tasty and perfect when served with a slice of crusty wholewheat or rye bread.

1 small onion
½ medium butternut squash
2 carrots, sliced
1 garlic clove, crushed
1 teaspoon (5 ml) grated fresh ginger
Pinch of freshly grated nutmeg (optional)
500 ml (16 fl oz) vegetable stock
1 tablespoon (15 ml) omega 3-rich oil or extra virgin olive oil
A little low-sodium salt and freshly ground black pepper

▸ Peel and chop the onion. Peel the butternut squash and cut the flesh into chunks.
▸ Place the vegetables, garlic, and grated ginger, optional nutmeg and vegetable stock in a large saucepan. Bring to the boil, lower the heat, cover and simmer for about 20 minutes until the vegetables are tender.
▸ Remove from the heat and liquidise with the oil until smooth, using a blender, food processor or a hand blender.
▸ Return to the saucepan to heat through. Season the soup with the low-sodium salt and freshly ground black pepper.

HEALTH STATISTICS
Butternut squash and carrots are rich in beta-carotene, which can help combat premature aging, heart disease and cancer. Butternut squash is also a useful source of the antioxidant vitamin C, which is needed for making collagen.

NUTRITIONAL ANALYSIS (PER SERVING):

Calories 115 kcal	Carbohydrate 15 g
Protein 1.7 g	Total sugars* 11 g
Fat 5.9 g	Fibre 3.5 g
Saturates 0.9 g	Salt 0.1 g

* total sugars includes sugars found naturally in foods

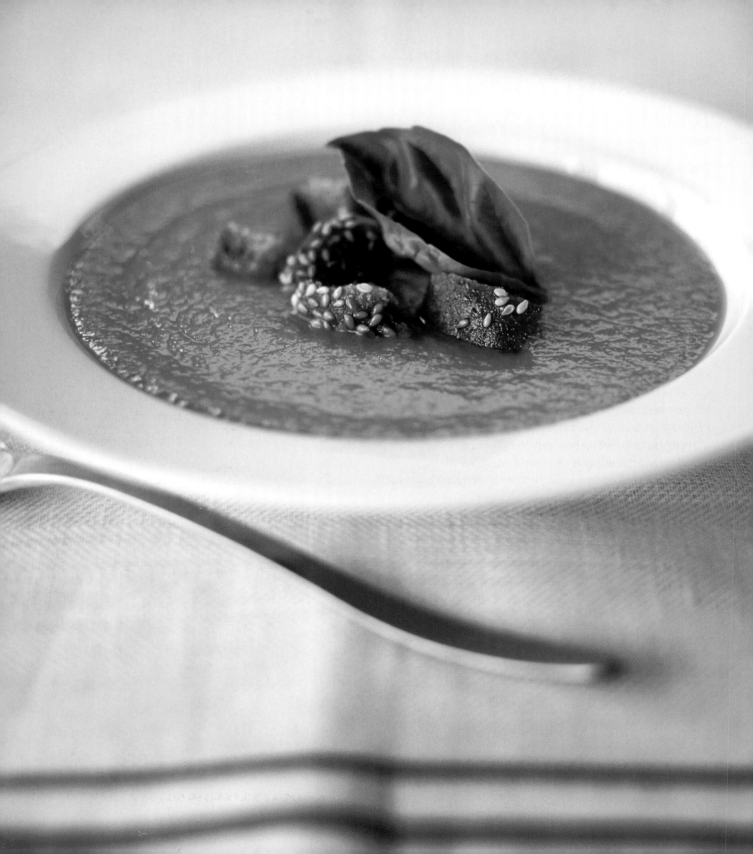

TOMATO SOUP WITH THYME AND TOASTED CROUTONS

MAKES 2 SERVINGS

Don't be tempted to open a tin or carton of tomato soup. This home-made version of an old favourite is well worth the extra bit of effort – and surprisingly easy, too. It's far lower in salt and sugar than bought varieties.

1 onion, chopped
1 garlic clove, crushed
1 tablespoon (15 ml) tomato purée
1 small carrot, diced
400 g tin chopped tomatoes
225 ml (8 fl oz) vegetable stock
1 teaspoon (5 ml) dried thyme

2 teaspoons (10 ml) cornflour,
mixed with a little water to a smooth paste
Squeeze of lemon juice
Freshly ground black pepper
1 thick slice wholegrain bread
1 tablespoon (15 ml) omega 3-rich oil or
extra virgin olive oil

▸ Place the onion, garlic, tomato purée, carrots, tinned tomatoes, vegetable stock and thyme in a large saucepan. Add the cornflour mixture and lemon juice. Bring to the boil, lower the heat, cover and simmer for 20–25 minutes.

▸ Meanwhile, toast the bread, then cut into 2-cm (³/₄-in) cubes.

▸ Remove the soup from the heat and liquidise with the oil and black pepper until smooth, using a blender, food processor or a hand blender.

▸ Ladle the soup into bowls and serve with a scattering of toasted croutons.

HEALTH STATISTICS
Tomatoes are a good source of beta-carotene, vitamins C and E, as well as numerous phytonutrients, including lycopene. This nutrient is responsible for the red colour in tomatoes and has been found to protect against heart disease and cancer. It is best absorbed when tomatoes are cooked.

NUTRITIONAL ANALYSIS (PER SERVING):

Calories 187 kcal	Carbohydrate 29 g
Protein 5.4 g	Total sugars* 15 g
Fat 6.5 g	Fibre 4.6 g
Saturates 0.9 g	Salt 0.5 g

* total sugars includes sugars found naturally in foods

PARSNIP AND CARROT SOUP

MAKES 4 SERVINGS

Here's a really simple way of using root vegetables. You can add other vegetables, such as swede and turnip too.

1 small onion, finely chopped
1 medium parsnip, peeled and sliced
2 carrots, sliced
500 ml (16 fl oz) vegetable stock

Freshly ground black pepper
1 tablespoon (15 ml) omega 3-rich oil
or extra virgin olive oil
2 tablespoons (30 ml) natural bio-yoghurt

▸ Place the vegetables and vegetable stock in a large saucepan. Bring to the boil, lower the heat, cover and simmer for about 20 minutes until the vegetables are tender.
▸ Allow the soup to cool a little. Stir in the oil and liquidise the soup, using a hand blender, food processor or blender. Season to taste with plenty of freshly ground black pepper.
▸ Ladle into bowls, then swirl a tablespoon of bio-yoghurt into the soup.

HEALTH STATISTICS
Parsnips are a rich source of complex carbohydrates and vitamin E. The carrots provide plenty of beta-carotene, vital for eyesight in dim light, healthy skin and immune function.

NUTRITIONAL ANALYSIS (PER SERVING):

Calories 159 kcal	Carbohydrate 21 g
Protein 4.1 g	Total sugars* 15 g
Fat 7.0 g	Fibre 5.8 g
Saturates 1.3 g	Salt 0.1 g

* total sugars includes sugars found naturally in foods

TUSCAN BEAN SOUP

MAKES 2 SERVINGS

This variation of minestrone soup is fantastically satisfying. You can substitute borlotti beans if you wish.

1 garlic clove, crushed
1 small onion, finely chopped
½ leek, finely chopped
1 carrot, peeled and chopped
400 g (14 oz) tin cannelloni beans, rinsed and drained
500 ml (16 fl oz) vegetable stock

1 bay leaf
½ teaspoon (2.5 ml) dried sage, crushed
2 tablespoons (30 ml) chopped fresh flat-leaf parsley, plus extra to garnish
Freshly ground black pepper
1 tablespoon (15 ml) omega 3-rich oil
or extra virgin olive oil

▸ Place the garlic, vegetables, beans, vegetable stock, bay leaf and sage in a large saucepan. Bring to the boil, lower the heat, cover and simmer for about 20 minutes until the vegetables are tender.
▸ Remove from the heat and remove the bay leaf. Stir in the fresh parsley. Season with freshly ground black pepper and ladle into warmed bowls. Scatter over the extra parsley and drizzle with the oil before serving.

HEALTH STATISTICS
This soup provides plenty of fibre (from the vegetables and the beans) which is important for efficient digestive function and colon health. The type of fibre provided by the beans also helps to lower blood cholesterol levels and protect against heart disease. They also supply good amounts of protein, complex carbohydrates, B vitamins and zinc.

NUTRITIONAL ANALYSIS (PER SERVING):

Calories 275 kcal	Carbohydrate 41 g
Protein 15 g	Total sugars* 7.3 g
Fat 6.9 g	Fibre 15 g
Saturates 1.1 g	Salt 0.1 g

* total sugars includes sugars found naturally in foods

ROASTED PUMPKIN SOUP

MAKES 2 SERVINGS

Don't buy pumpkin only for Halloween. Its available for several months over winter and this soup is an ideal way of reaping its health benefits.

350 g (10 oz) pumpkin flesh, cubed
2 garlic cloves, halved
1 tablespoon (15 ml) olive oil
1 onion, chopped
1 clove of garlic, chopped
1/2 teaspoon (2.5 ml) grated fresh ginger
1 teaspoon (5 ml) ground coriander
500 ml (16 fl oz) vegetable stock
Freshly ground black pepper

▸ Preheat the oven to 200°C/400°F/Gas mark 6.
▸ Put the pumpkin and garlic cloves in a roasting tin and toss with the olive oil. Roast in the oven for 30 minutes.
▸ Put the garlic, pumpkin, ginger, ground coriander and stock in a large saucepan. Bring to the boil, then reduce the heat and simmer for 10 minutes.
▸ Liquidise the soup using a hand blender or conventional blender. Add a little more water or stock if you want a thinner consistency. Season to taste with freshly ground black pepper.

HEALTH STATISTICS
Pumpkin is super-rich in the phytonutrient alpha-carotene, which helps prevent cancer. It is also rich in vitamin E, beta-carotene and vitamin C. Both alpha- and beta-carotene can be converted in the body to vitamin A.

NUTRITIONAL ANALYSIS (PER SERVING):

Calories 99 kcal	Carbohydrate 9.8 g
Protein 2.1 g	Total sugars* 7.2 g
Fat 6.0 g	Fibre 2.8 g
Saturates 1.0 g	Salt 0.1 g

* total sugars includes sugars found naturally in foods

THAI PRAWN AND MUSHROOM SOUP

MAKES 2 SERVINGS

This beautiful-looking soup is perfect for serving to guests at dinner parties. You can adjust the amount of chilli according to your taste.

1 shallot (or onion), chopped
2-cm (³/₄-in) piece fresh root ginger, chopped
1 tablespoon (15 ml) chilli sauce
500 ml (16 fl oz) vegetable stock
1 lemongrass stalk, lightly crushed

8 tiger prawns, shelled, deveined
125 g (4oz) shitake mushrooms
Juice of 1 lime
Small handful fresh coriander
leaves, roughly chopped

▶ Place the shallots, ginger, chilli sauce and stock in a large pan. Bring to the boil, then reduce the heat and simmer for 10 minutes. Add the mushrooms and prawns and cook for a few minutes. Add the lime juice then ladle into bowls. Scatter over the coriander leaves.

HEALTH STATISTICS
Shitake mushrooms have powerful immunity and healing properties and are also believed to help beat numerous conditions, from colds and flu to gastrointestinal problems. They supply good amounts of B vitamins, magnesium, iron and potassium.

NUTRITIONAL ANALYSIS (PER SERVING):
Calories 59 kcal   Carbohydrate 9.4 g
Protein 5.1 g   Total sugars* 1.7 g
Fat 0.3 g   Fibre 0.3 g
Saturates 0.1 g   Salt 1.2 g
* total sugars includes sugars found naturally in foods

CABBAGE SOUP

MAKES 2 SERVINGS

Most people only ever serve cabbage as an accompanying vegetable. Here's an ingenious and simple way of serving it. Use green cabbage or Savoy cabbage when in season.

¹/₂ green cabbage
1 garlic clove, crushed
1 carrot, sliced
1 small turnip, peeled and chopped
1 medium potato, peeled and chopped

1 bouquet garni
500 ml (16 fl oz) vegetable stock
Freshly ground black pepper
1 tablespoon (15 ml) omega 3-rich oil
or extra virgin olive oil

▶ Discard the outer tough leaves of the cabbage, cut out the large veins then shred the leaves. Place the prepared vegetables, garlic, bouquet garni and vegetable stock in a large saucepan. Bring to the boil, lower the heat, cover and simmer gently for about 25 minutes until the vegetables are tender.
▶ Remove from the heat and remove the bouquet garni. Season with freshly ground black pepper, stir in the oil and ladle in individual bowls.

HEALTH STATISTICS
Cabbage contains antioxidant vitamin C, which helps boost the immune system, and beta-carotene, which helps fight cancer. It also provides glucosinolates, plant chemicals that help protect the body from cancer.

NUTRITIONAL ANALYSIS (PER SERVING):
Calories 153 kcal   Carbohydrate 22 g
Protein 3.7 g   Total sugars* 9.0 g
Fat 6.3 g   Fibre 5.0 g
Saturates 0.9 g   Salt 0.2 g
* total sugars includes sugars found naturally in foods

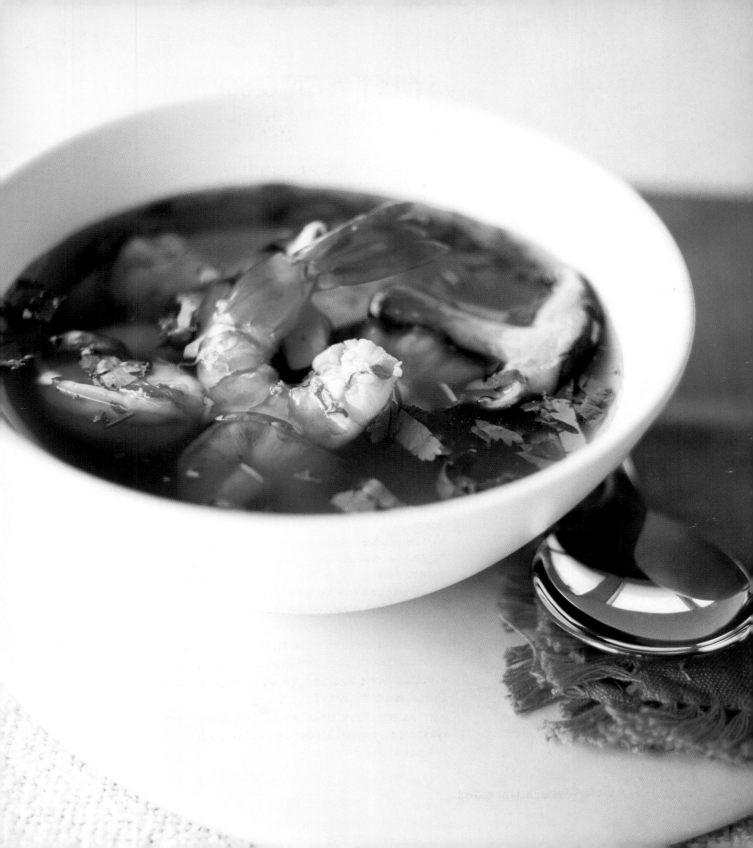

SWEET POTATO SOUP

MAKES 2 SERVINGS

This simple soup is one of my favourite mid-week quick meals. Its delicious and really satisfying served with a simple salad.

250 g (9 oz) sweet potatoes, peeled and chopped
1 small onion, sliced
500 ml (16 fl oz) vegetable stock
1 tablespoon (15 ml) omega 3-rich oil or extra virgin olive oil
Freshly ground black pepper

▸ Put the potatoes, onions and stock in a large saucepan. Bring to the boil, then reduce the heat and simmer for 15 minutes or until the vegetables are tender.
▸ Stir in the oil and liquidise the soup using a hand blender, food processor or blender. Season to taste with plenty of freshly ground black pepper.

HEALTH STATISTICS
Sweet potatoes are rich in beta-carotene, an antioxidant that helps fight cancer, and which the body also converts to vitamin A. In addition, it is rich in vitamin E, which is vital for healthy skin.

NUTRITIONAL ANALYSIS (PER SERVING):

Calories 185 kcal	Carbohydrate 33 g
Protein 2.4 g	Total sugars* 11 g
Fat 6.0 g	Fibre 4.1 g
Saturates 0.9 g	Salt 0.1 g

* total sugars includes sugars found naturally in foods

AL FRESCO TOMATO SOUP

MAKES 2 SERVINGS

This soup is perfect when tomatoes are plentiful and cheap. It requires no cooking so all the nutrients are retained in the soup.

675 g (1 ½ lb) tomatoes, skinned and quartered
2 garlic cloves, roughly sliced
½ small red onion, roughly chopped
2 tablespoons (30 ml) tomato purée
125 ml (4 fl oz) tomato juice (low salt)
1 tablespoon (15 ml) extra virgin olive oil
2 tablespoons (30 ml) lemon juice
A little low-sodium salt and freshly ground black pepper, to taste
A few basil or tarragon leaves, roughly torn

▸ Place all the ingredients except the fresh herbs in a food processor or blender and blend until smooth. Add a little cold water to thin it, if necessary. Taste the soup and adjust the seasoning with a little more lemon juice, low-sodium salt or pepper.
▸ Pour into a bowl, cover and chill for at least an hour before serving. Stir before serving, sprinkled with the torn basil leaves or tarragon.

HEALTH STATISTICS
This soup is super-rich in vitamin C, a terrific immunity booster that's also good for your skin. The tomatoes are also rich in beta-carotene and lycopene, both powerful anti-cancer nutrients.

NUTRITIONAL ANALYSIS (PER SERVING):

Calories 138 kcal	Carbohydrate 17 g
Protein 4.0 g	Total sugars* 16 g
Fat 6.6 g	Fibre 4.6 g
Saturates 1.1 g	Salt 0.5 g

* total sugars includes sugars found naturally in foods

WATERCRESS SOUP

MAKES 2 SERVINGS

Watercress is not only for salads. It also works well in soup, where it adds
a wonderful, intense colour and a hint of peppery flavour.

1 small onion, chopped
1 small potato, peeled and chopped
1 bunch watercress, roughly chopped
250 ml (8 fl oz) vegetable stock
250 ml (8 fl oz) skimmed milk, or non-dairy milk
1 tablespoon (15 ml) omega 3-rich oil or extra virgin olive oil
A little low-sodium salt and freshly ground black pepper
2 tablespoons (30 ml) plain bio-yoghurt to serve

▸ Place the vegetables and vegetable stock in a large saucepan. Bring to the boil, lower
the heat, cover and simmer for about 15–20 minutes until the potatoes are tender.
▸ Allow the soup to cool a little. Stir in the milk and oil and liquidise the soup, using a
hand blender, food processor or blender. Season to taste with plenty of freshly ground
black pepper.
▸ Ladle into bowls, then swirl a tablespoon of bio-yoghurt into the soup.

HEALTH STATISTICS
Watercress is rich in glucosinolates, plant
chemicals that boost the activity of anti-cancer
enzymes. It also contains antioxidant vitamins,
beta-carotene and vitamin C, which help
promote good immunity, as well as vitamin B6,
iron and folate.

NUTRITIONAL ANALYSIS (PER SERVING):

Calories 186 kcal	Carbohydrate 24 g
Protein 9.0 g	Total sugars* 11 g
Fat 6.7 g	Fibre 1.6 g
Saturates 1.3 g	Salt 0.3 g

* total sugars includes sugars found naturally in foods

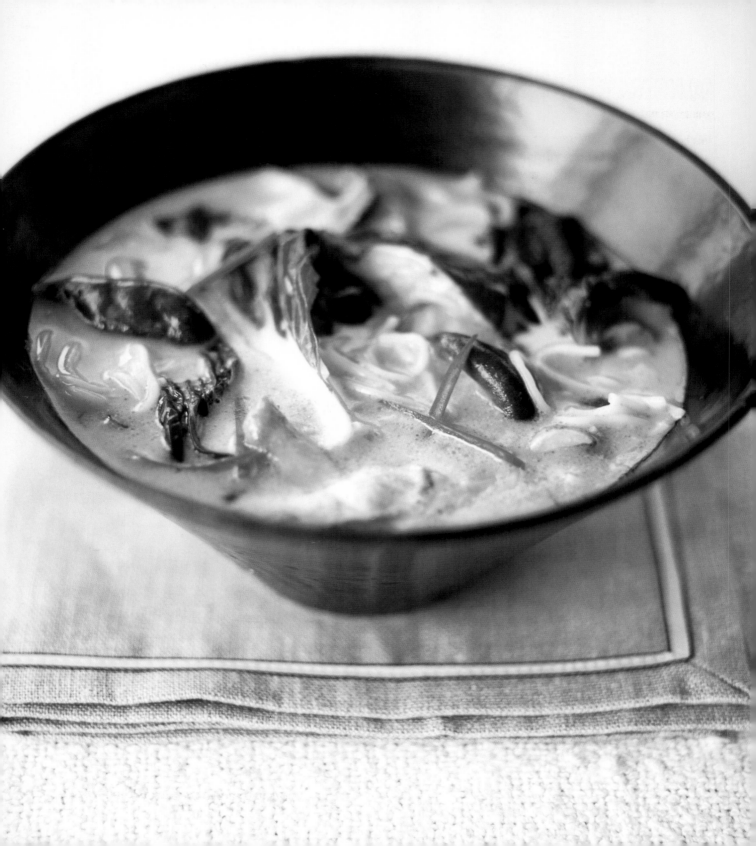

LAKSA

MAKES 2 SERVINGS

This Malaysian soup is great to serve to non-vegetarian guests who will
be pleasantly surprised that meat-free dishes can taste this good. For a less
authentic dish, you can substitute green cabbage for the pak choi.

60 g (2 oz) rice noodles
1 tablespoon (15 ml) olive oil
2 teaspoons (10 ml) Thai paste
1/2 small red chilli, deseeded and finely sliced
125 g (4 oz) shitake mushrooms, sliced
200 ml (7 fl oz) coconut milk
300 ml (1/2 pint) water
1 bok choi (sometimes called pak choi), trimmed and roughly chopped
60 g (2 oz) baby sweetcorn
A little low-sodium salt and freshly ground black pepper
Small handful of fresh coriander leaves, roughly chopped

▸ Put the noodles in a bowl and cover with boiling water. Leave to soak for 10 minutes,
then drain.
▸ Meanwhile, heat the oil in a large pan, add the Thai paste and stir for a few moments.
Add the chilli and mushrooms and cook for 1–2 minutes. Add the coconut milk and
water. Bring to the boil, then reduce the heat and simmer for 5 minutes.
▸ Add the bok choi and continue cooking for a further 5 minutes. Add the
sweetcorn and noodles and cook for a further 2 minutes. Season with the low-sodium
salt and freshly ground black pepper. Ladle into bowls and top with a generous
amount of coriander.

HEALTH STATISTICS

This soup is a good source of fibre. Bok choi,
a popular green vegetable in Asia (now widely
available in supermarkets) contains anti-cancer
phytochemicals, including flavanoids and
isothiocyanates. These help stimulate the body's
detoxification system and block the action of
cancer-causing substances. The vegetable is also
a good source of calcium, folate and potassium.

NUTRITIONAL ANALYSIS (PER SERVING):

Calories 252 kcal	Carbohydrate 41 g
Protein 5.0 g	Total sugars* 8.6 g
Fat 7.4 g	Fibre 2.4 g
Saturates 1.1 g	Salt 0.5 g

* total sugars includes sugars found naturally in foods

CHAPTER 10
DESSERTS

STRAWBERRIES AND RASPBERRIES WITH TOFU 'CREAM'

MAKES 2 SERVINGS

This simple combination of summer fruits is delicious served with this low-fat alternative to dairy cream. It's also good with plain bio-yoghurt mixed with a few drops of vanilla extract.

175 g (6 oz) strawberries, halved
125 g (4 oz) raspberries
125 ml (4 fl oz) apple or orange juice

FOR THE TOFU 'CREAM':
100 g (3½ oz) silken tofu, drained
Juice and zest of ½ small orange
1 teaspoon (5 ml) lemon juice
1 teaspoon (5 ml) clear honey

▸ Place the fruit in a medium-sized bowl. Pour over the fruit juice and turn gently. Ideally leave for 30 minutes in the fridge to allow the flavours to infuse.
▸ Meanwhile make the tofu 'cream'. Place the 'cream' ingredients in a blender or food processor. Cover and chill in the fridge until needed.
▸ Serve the fruit with the 'cream'.

HEALTH STATISTICS
Both strawberries and raspberries are packed with vitamin C, which helps strengthen collagen as well as fight free radicals responsible for aging. They also contain high levels of the antioxidant ellagic acid, which can help combat cancer, and anthocyanins, which promote healthy skin. Tofu is rich in protein and calcium as well as phytoestrogens, which makes it useful for helping combat some of the symptoms of the menopause, such as hot flushes. Other substances (called protease inhibitors) can help protect against cancer.

NUTRITIONAL ANALYSIS (PER SERVING):

Calories 116 kcal	Carbohydrate 19 g
Protein 5.8 g	Total sugars* 19 g
Fat 2.4 g	Fibre 2.5 g
Saturates 0.3 g	Salt 0.1 g

* total sugars includes sugars found naturally in foods

EXOTIC FRUIT SALAD WITH ALMONDS

MAKES 2 SERVINGS

You can prepare this fruit salad in advance and leave it in the fridge for up to a day. Don't add the banana until just before serving to prevent it turning brown.

125 ml (4 fl oz) orange juice
1 passion fruit
½ mango
½ fresh pineapple
(or approx 4 rings of tinned pineapple)
1 nectarine
1 banana
30 g (1 oz) flaked toasted almonds

▸ Halve the passion fruit, scoop out the seeds and add them to the orange juice in a large bowl.
▸ Slice through the mango either side of the stone. Peel, then cut the flesh into cubes.
▸ Cut the pineapple into 4 x 1-cm (½-in) rounds, then cut each round into quarters. Slice the nectarine and banana. Add the prepared fruit to the bowl and turn gently in the juice.
▸ Leave the fruit salad in the fridge to allow the flavours to blend. Scatter over the flaked toasted almonds before serving.

HEALTH STATISTICS
This salad provides lots of fibre, vitamin C, beta-carotene and potassium. Mangos are one of the few fruit sources of vitamin E, an important antioxidant that helps to fight damaging free radicals in the body

NUTRITIONAL ANALYSIS (PER SERVING):

Calories 265 kcal	Carbohydrate 42 g
Protein 6.1 g	Total sugars* 41 g
Fat 9.1 g	Fibre 5.3 g
Saturates 0.8 g	Salt 0.1 g

* total sugars includes sugars found naturally in foods

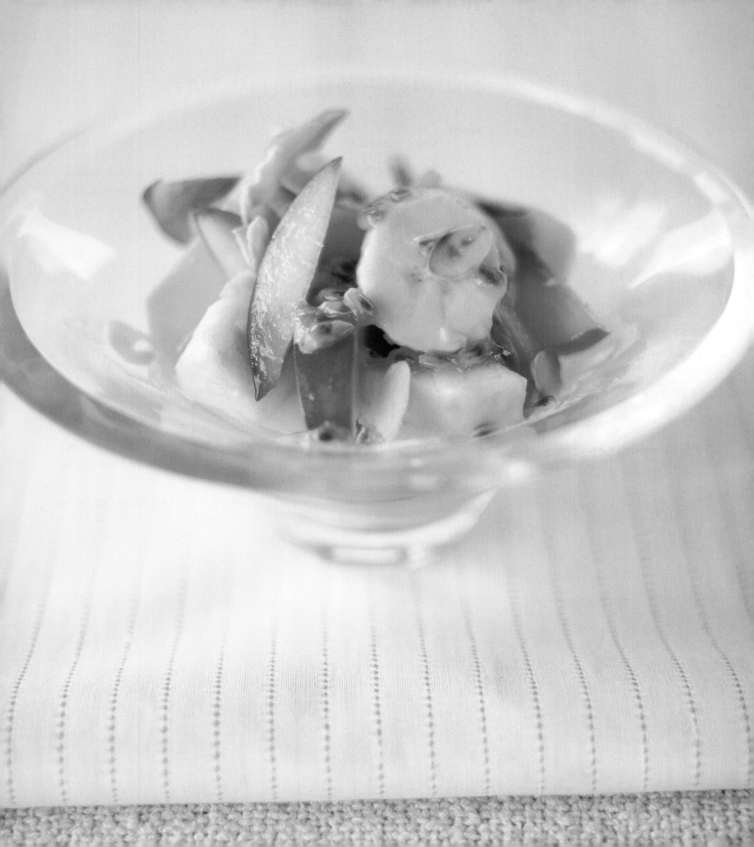

POACHED PLUMS WITH GINGER AND YOGHURT

MAKES 2 SERVINGS

Choose ripe but firm plums for this recipe. Purple plums are delicious poached this way, but other varieties, such as Victorias, also work well. You can make a larger quantity and keep the remaining portions in the fridge for up to 3 days.

125 g (4 fl oz) water
1 tablespoon (15 ml) clear honey
225g g (8 oz) purple plums
2.5-cm (1-in) piece root ginger, chopped
Plain bio-yoghurt to serve

▸ Place the water and honey in a saucepan and bring slowly to the boil, stirring occasionally until the honey has dissolved.
▸ Halve the plums and remove the stones. Add them to the honey liquor with the chopped ginger. Simmer gently for 10 minutes until the plums are tender.
▸ Cover and chill in the fridge until required. Serve the plums and their liquor with plain bio-yoghurt.

HEALTH STATISTICS
Purple plums are a good source of fibre and antioxidants, in particular hydroxycinnamic acid, which can help reduce the risk of colon cancer. Stewing doesn't destroy the antioxidant benefits.

NUTRITIONAL ANALYSIS (PER SERVING):

Calories 65 kcal	Carbohydrate 16 g
Protein 0.7 g	Total sugars* 16 g
Fat 0.1 g	Fibre 1.8 g
Saturates 0 g	Salt 0.1 g

* total sugars includes sugars found naturally in foods

DRIED FRUIT COMPOTE IN JASMINE TEA

MAKES 2 SERVINGS

You can use ready-made mixtures of dried fruit or assemble your own mix from prunes, figs, apricots, mango or apple rings. This recipe can be prepared in advance and kept in the fridge for up to 3 days.

1 teaspoon (5 ml) jasmine tea leaves
125 g (4 oz) dried fruit mixture
Zest and juice of 1 orange
1 cinnamon stick

▸ Place the tea leaves in an infuser or tie in a muslin bag. Place in a saucepan, then add the dried fruits, orange zest and cinnamon. Pour enough boiling water over the fruit to cover. Bring to the boil, then reduce the heat and simmer for about 15 minutes until the fruit is tender. Add the orange juice and discard the tea leaves and cinnamon stick.
▸ Leave to cool and keep covered in the fridge for at least 2 hours (or preferably overnight) until you are ready to serve.

HEALTH STATISTICS
Dried fruit is a concentrated source of soluble fibre, which helps balance blood sugar levels, reduce cholesterol levels and promote healthy digestion. Dried apricots are rich in beta-carotene and iron; figs are rich in calcium and prunes have one of the highest antioxidant scores of all fruits.

NUTRITIONAL ANALYSIS (PER SERVING):

Calories 108 kcal	Carbohydrate 25 g
Protein 2.7 g	Total sugars* 25 g
Fat 0.4 g	Fibre 4.0 g
Saturates 0 g	Salt 0.1 g

* total sugars includes sugars found naturally in foods

AUTUMN FRUIT SALAD

MAKES 2 SERVINGS

This simple dish of seasonal fresh fruit is also good with dried fruit – try adding a few dried apple rings or pears and leave to soak in the orange juice-honey liquor for an hour or longer before serving.

1 pear
2 small Cox apples
1 banana, peeled and sliced
4 tablespoons (60 ml) orange juice
1 tablespoon (15 ml) acacia (or clear) honey

▸ Cut the pear and apples into quarters, then slice thinly. Slice the banana. Place the prepared fruit in a large bowl.
▸ Add the orange juice and honey and turn the fruit to mix. Cover and chill until you are ready to serve.

HEALTH STATISTICS
Apples are rich in fibre, potassium and the flavanoid, quercetin, which has anti-cancer and anti-inflammatory properties. Pears are also good sources of fibre and contain hydroxycinnamic acids, which help fight cancer, especially of the colon.

NUTRITIONAL ANALYSIS (PER SERVING):

Calories 161 kcal	Carbohydrate 40 g
Protein 1.5 g	Total sugars* 39 g
Fat 0.3 g	Fibre 4.1 g
Saturates 0.1 g	Salt 0.1 g

* total sugars includes sugars found naturally in foods

Strawberries are packed with vitamin C – one serving of this dish gives you 100 per cent of your daily requirement of this immunity-boosting vitamin. Both strawberries and blueberries contain ellagic acid, a phytonutrient shown to help fight cancer and destroy toxins absorbed from pollution and cigarette smoke. Blueberries, ranked one of the most nutritious fruit of all for their antioxidant power, contain anthocyanins, which may help delay aging.

NUTRITIONAL ANALYSIS (PER SERVING):

Calories 135 kcal	Carbohydrate 26 g
Protein 6.0 g	Total sugars* 26 g
Fat 1.2 g	Fibre 2.8 g
Saturates 0.7 g	Salt 0.1 g

* total sugars includes sugars found naturally in foods

BLUEBERRIES AND STRAWBERRIES WITH VANILLA YOGHURT

MAKES 2 SERVINGS

If I had to choose my perfect dessert, this would be it. I love the combination of colours and flavours. This dessert is a real treat when berries are in season.

150 g (5 oz) strawberries
150 g (5 oz) blueberries
2 teaspoons (10 ml) caster sugar

200 ml (7 fl oz) plain live bio-yoghurt
2 teaspoons (10 ml) acacia honey
A few drops of vanilla extract

▸ Wash and hull the strawberries. Halve or quarter the fruits. Place in a large bowl with the blueberries. Sprinkle over the sugar and turn gently. Combine the yoghurt, honey and vanilla in a separate bowl. Arrange the berries on two plates and spoon the vanilla yoghurt on top or on the side.

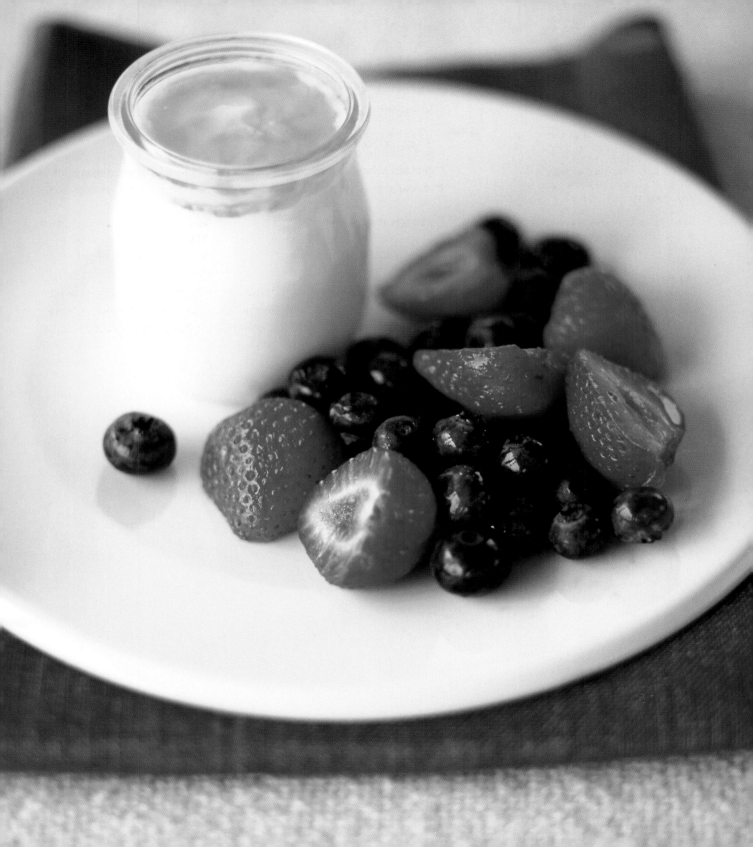

REAL STRAWBERRY YOGHURT

MAKES 2 SERVINGS

It's so easy making real fruit yoghurt at home from fresh seasonal fruit and plain yoghurt. If you toast a larger batch of nuts and keep it in a sealed container, you will have a ready supply to sprinkle on yoghurt desserts, as well as cereals and salads.

1 tablespoon (15 ml) hazelnuts
1 tablespoon (15 ml) flaked almonds
1 tablespoon (15 ml) porridge oats
250 ml (8 fl oz) plain live bio-yoghurt
175 g (6 oz) strawberries

▸ Pre-heat the oven to 190°C/375°F/Gas Mark 5.
▸ Spread the nuts on a baking tray, then lightly toast in the oven for 5–7 minutes until they turn pale golden brown. Keep a careful eye on them in case they over-brown. Allow to cool, then mix with the oats.
▸ Wash, hull and quarter the strawberries.
▸ Put the yoghurt in a bowl, then add the strawberries, nuts and oats. Mix to combine and then serve.

HEALTH STATISTICS
Live bio-yoghurt provides lots of calcium, which not only helps promote strong bones but can help weight loss. It also contains friendly bacteria, which encourage healthy digestion, reduce bloating and boost immunity. The strawberries add vitamin C and the nuts provide heart-healthy fats, vitamin E and extra fibre.

NUTRITIONAL ANALYSIS (PER SERVING):

Calories 196 kcal	Carbohydrate 21 g
Protein 9.7 g	Total sugars* 15 g
Fat 8.8 g	Fibre 2.3 g
Saturates 1.4 g	Salt 0.2 g

* total sugars includes sugars found naturally in foods

MELON AND MANGO SKEWERS

MAKES 2 SERVINGS

These skewers are a fun way of serving fruit and perfect for picnics.
For a treat, serve them with chocolate sauce, made by simply melting
dark chocolate containing 70 per cent cocoa solids.

2 apricots
½ cantaloupe melon
1 nectarine
1 small mango, peeled and stoned

▸ Halve the apricots and remove the stones. Cut the melon in half and scoop out the
seeds. Either scoop out the flesh using a melon baller, or slice and then cut into cubes.
Slice the nectarine and cut the mango flesh into chunks.

▸ Thread the fruit onto 4 wooden skewers; making sure that each has a mixture of fruit.
Serve immediately.

HEALTH STATISTICS
This dessert is packed with beta-carotene – the
apricots, cantaloupe melon, necatarine and
mango are all rich sources of this vitamin, which
helps protect against certain cancers as well as
defend the skin against sun damage.

NUTRITIONAL ANALYSIS (PER SERVING):

Calories 114 kcal	Carbohydrate 26 g
Protein 2.8 g	Total sugars* 26 g
Fat 0.4 g	Fibre 5.0 g
Saturates 0.1 g	Salt 0.1 g

* total sugars includes sugars found naturally in foods

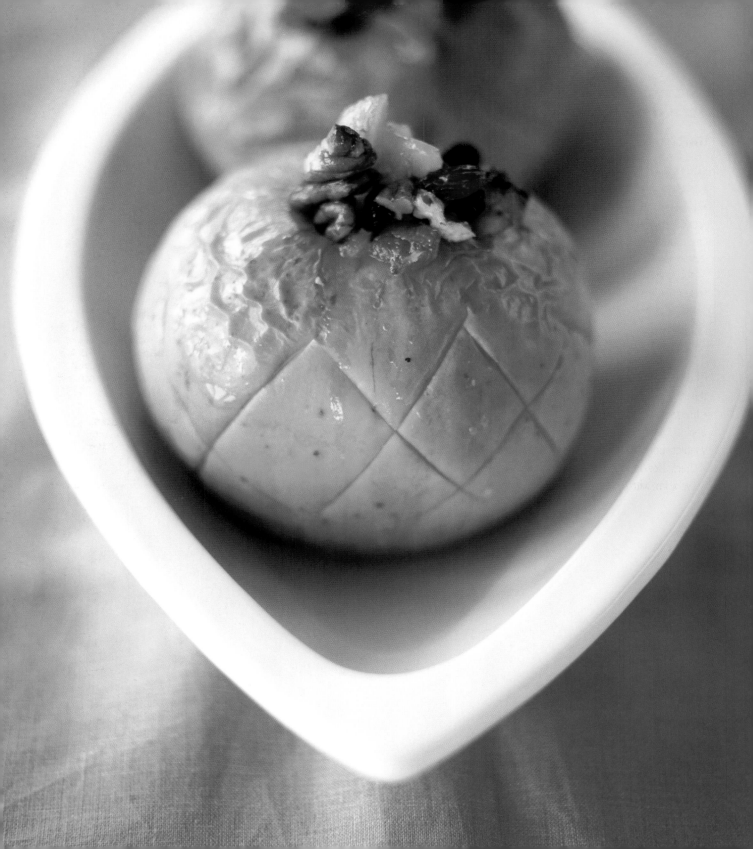

BAKED APPLES WITH FRUIT AND NUTS

MAKES 2 SERVINGS

This version of one my favourite comfort foods is made healthier with the addition of apricots and nuts and also by replacing the usual sugar with a little honey. You can substitute dates or dried figs for the raisins and apricots if you want, or use other types of nuts instead of pecans.

2 Bramley cooking apples
1 tablespoon (15 ml) raisins or sultanas
6–8 ready-to-eat dried apricots, chopped
2 teaspoons (10 ml) clear honey
1 tablespoon (15 ml) pecans, chopped

▸ Pre-heat the oven to 190°C/375°F/Gas Mark 5.
▸ Remove the core from the apples. Using a sharp knife, lightly score the skin around the middle, just enough to pierce the skin.
▸ In a small bowl, combine the dried fruit, honey and pecans. Fill the cavities of the apples, then place them in a baking dish. They should fit snugly side by side. Add 2 tablespoons of water, cover loosely with foil then bake for 45– 60 minutes.
▸ Check a few times during cooking, adding a little extra water if the dish becomes dry. Serve warm with plain live bio-yoghurt.

HEALTH STATISTICS
Bramley apples contain the antioxidant quercetin – which can help fight cancer – as well as good amounts of vitamin C and potassium. The apricots provide beta-carotene, while the raisins provide extra fibre and antioxidants. The pecan nuts give you essential omega-3 oils and vitamin E.

NUTRITIONAL ANALYSIS (PER SERVING):

Calories 215 kcal	Carbohydrate 41 g
Protein 2.7 g	Total sugars* 41 g
Fat 5.7 g	Fibre 4.9 g
Saturates 0.4 g	Salt 0.1 g

* total sugars includes sugars found naturally in foods

STRAWBERRY AND RHUBARB CRUMBLE

MAKES 4 SERVINGS

**This crumble is packed with the flavours of summer – divine!
Choose tender pink rhubarb when it is in season.**

2–3 stalks young rhubarb
125 g (4 oz) fresh strawberries
2 tablespoons (30 ml) water
4 tablespoons (60 ml) clear honey
40g (1 1/2 oz) flaked almonds, crushed

40 g (1 1/2 oz) oats
15 g (1/2 oz) millet flakes
15 g (1/2 oz) rice flour
40g (1 1/2 oz) olive oil spread

▸ Pre-heat the oven to 190°C/375°F/Gas Mark 5.
▸ Trim the rhubarb and cut into 2.5-cm (1-in) lengths. Hull the strawberries and cut any large fruit in half. Put the prepared fruit into an ovenproof dish. In a saucepan, melt 2 tablespoons (30 ml) of the honey with the water over a low heat. Pour over the fruit and mix together.
▸ Place the flaked almonds, oats, rice flour, olive oil spread and the remaining honey in a bowl and mix together with your fingers until you have a sticky crumb mixture. Alternatively, put in a food processor and pulse until the mixture forms fine crumbs.
▸ Spread the oat crumble over the fruit and bake in the oven for about 20 minutes until the topping is golden.

HEALTH STATISTICS

Both the rhubarb and strawberries are good sources of immunity-boosting vitamin C and other compounds that help prevent cancer. Rhubarb is high in fibre, helpful for lowering cholesterol and preventing heart disease. It also contains oxalic acid, which helps the body's natural detoxification process. The topping contains almonds for extra protein, calcium and heart-healthy monounsaturated oils.

NUTRITIONAL ANALYSIS (PER SERVING):

Calories 238 kcal	Carbohydrate 28 g
Protein 4.4 g	Total sugars* 14 g
Fat 13 g	Fibre 2.3 g
Saturates 1.6 g	Salt 0.2 g

* total sugars includes sugars found naturally in foods

STRAWBERRY AND MANGO SALAD WITH LIME

MAKES 2 SERVINGS

This beautiful combination of fresh fruits is one of my favourites.
Serve it at room temperature for the flavours to come through.

225 g (8 oz) strawberries
1 small ripe mango
Grated zest and juice of 1 lime
2 teaspoons (10 ml) clear honey

▸ Wash, hull and halve the strawberries. Slice through the mango either side of the stone, then peel and cut the flesh into cubes. Place the fruit in a serving bowl.
▸ Grate the zest from the lime and add to the fruit. Squeeze the juice then put in a small saucepan with the honey. Heat gently, stirring, just until the honey has dissolved. Allow to cool.
▸ Pour the cooled lime juice over the fruit and toss gently.

HEALTH STATISTICS

Mangos are the best fruit source of the antioxidant beta-carotene, which helps promote healthy skin and improve its elasticity. It also provides vitamin C, vitamin E and potassium. Strawberries are super-rich in vitamin C, which is good for strengthening blood vessels and protecting against free radical damage.

NUTRITIONAL ANALYSIS (PER SERVING):

Calories 98 kcal	Carbohydrate 24 g
Protein 1.5 g	Total sugars* 24 g
Fat 0.3 g	Fibre 3.2 g
Saturates 0.1 g	Salt 0.1 g

* total sugars includes sugars found naturally in foods

CHAPTER 11
DRINKS AND SMOOTHIES

RASPBERRY AND BLUEBERRY SMOOTHIE

MAKES 2 DRINKS

125 g (4 oz) raspberries
125 g (4 oz) blueberries
1 small banana, peeled and cut into chunks
125 ml (4 fl oz) fresh orange juice
A cupful of crushed ice

▸ Place the ingredients in a smoothie maker, blender or food processor and blend until smooth and frothy. Serve immediately.

HEALTH STATISTICS
Blueberries and raspberries are packed with immunity-boosting vitamin C and anthocyanins, which have a myriad of health benefits, including protection from heart disease and cancer and against degenerative eye disease and dementia.

NUTRITIONAL ANALYSIS (PER SERVING):

Calories 99 kcal	Carbohydrate 23 g
Protein 2.4 g	Total sugars* 22 g
Fat 0.5 g	Fibre 4.1 g
Saturates 0.1 g	Salt 0.1 g

* total sugars includes sugars found naturally in foods

RED BERRY SMOOTHIE

MAKES 2 DRINKS

About 5–6 ice cubes, crushed
85 g (3 oz) strawberries
60 g (2 oz) raspberries
1 banana
200 ml (7 fl oz) orange juice

▸ Place the ingredients in a smoothie maker, blender or food processor and blend until smooth and frothy. Serve immediately.

HEALTH STATISTICS
Strawberries and raspberries are terrific sources of vitamin C. One drink gives you 100 per cent of the daily requirement for this vitamin (60mg). They also contain ellagic acid, a phytonutrient that fights cancer.

NUTRITIONAL ANALYSIS (PER SERVING):

Calories 102 kcal	Carbohydrate 24 g
Protein 1.9 g	Total sugars* 23 g
Fat 0.4 g	Fibre 1.9 g
Saturates 0.1 g	Salt 0.1 g

* total sugars includes sugars found naturally in foods

MELON WHIZ

MAKES 2 DRINKS

½ cantaloupe melon
120 ml (4 fl oz) orange juice
1 tablespoon (15 ml) lemon juice

▸ Place the ingredients in a smoothie maker, blender or food processor and blend until smooth and frothy. Serve immediately.

HEALTH STATISTICS
Cantaloupe melon is packed with beta-carotene, which benefits your skin and protects against many cancers. Orange and lemon juice add extra vitamin C.

NUTRITIONAL ANALYSIS (PER SERVING):

Calories 60 kcal	Carbohydrate 14 g
Protein 1.5 g	Total sugars* 14 g
Fat 0.3 g	Fibre 2.1 g
Saturates 0 g	Salt 0.1 g

* total sugars includes sugars found naturally in foods

CITRUS REFRESHER

MAKES 2 DRINKS

1 pink grapefruit, peeled and divided into segments
2 oranges, peeled and divided into segments
2 tablespoons (30 ml) lemon juice
1 tablespoon (15 ml) honey

▶ Place the grapefruit, oranges in a smoothie maker, blender or food processor and process until smooth. Serve immediately. Alternatively, you can process the fruit in a citrus juicer then combine with the lemon juice and honey.

CRANBERRY SMOOTHIE

MAKES 2 DRINKS

A small cupful of crushed ice
250 ml (8 fl oz) cranberry juice drink
60 g (2 oz) raspberries
1 carton (150 g) natural yoghurt

▶ Place the ingredients in a smoothie maker, blender or food processor and blend until smooth and frothy. Serve immediately.

BETA-POWER

MAKES 2 DRINKS

A small cupful of crushed ice
1/2 mango, peeled, stone removed and diced
120 ml (4 fl oz) carrot juice
125 g (4 oz) strawberries
1/2 red pepper

▶ Place the ingredients in a smoothie maker, blender or food processor and blend until smooth and frothy. Serve immediately.

WATERMELON ZINGER

MAKES 2 DRINKS

A cupful of crushed ice
2 slices watermelon (about 300 g/10 oz flesh)
Juice of 1 orange
125 g (4 oz) strawberries

▶ Scrape out the seeds from the watermelon. Place the flesh with the other ingredients in a smoothie maker, blender or food processor and blend until smooth and frothy. Serve immediately.

PICK-ME-UP PUNCH

MAKES 2 DRINKS

125 g (4 oz) blueberries
1 peach, stone removed and chopped
120 ml (4 fl oz) apple juice
85 ml (3 fl oz) natural yoghurt or silken tofu
5–6 ice cubes

▶ Place the ingredients in a smoothie maker, blender or food processor and blend until smooth and frothy. Serve immediately.

ZESTY ZINGER

MAKES 2 DRINKS

120 ml (5 fl oz) orange juice
120 ml (5 fl oz) pineapple juice
85 ml (3 fl oz) cranberry juice drink
1/2–1 teaspoon (2.5–5 ml) finely grated fresh ginger

▶ Pour the juices into a large glass and mix well. Stir in the grated ginger.

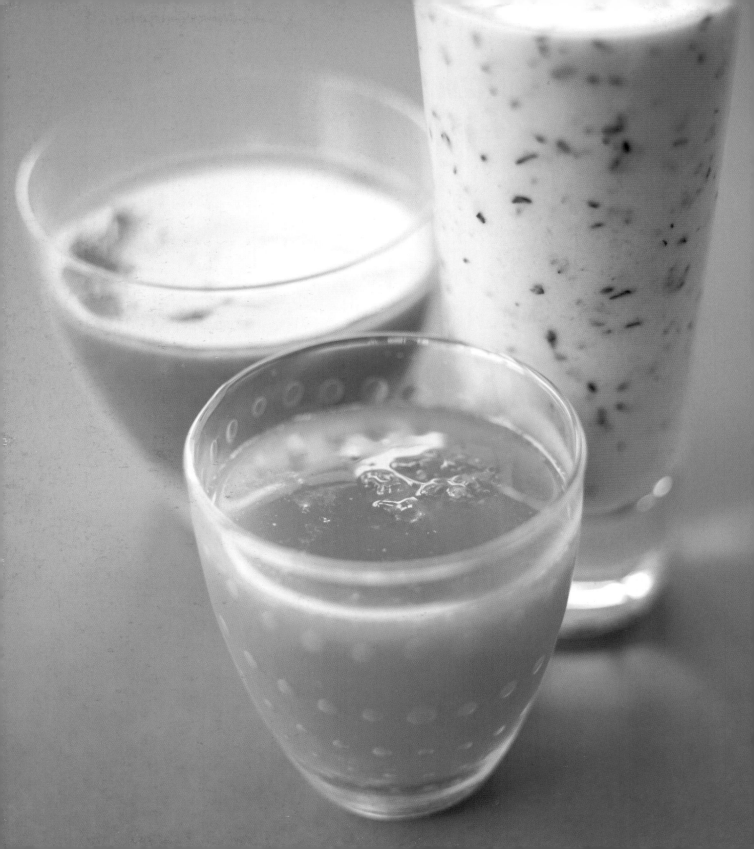

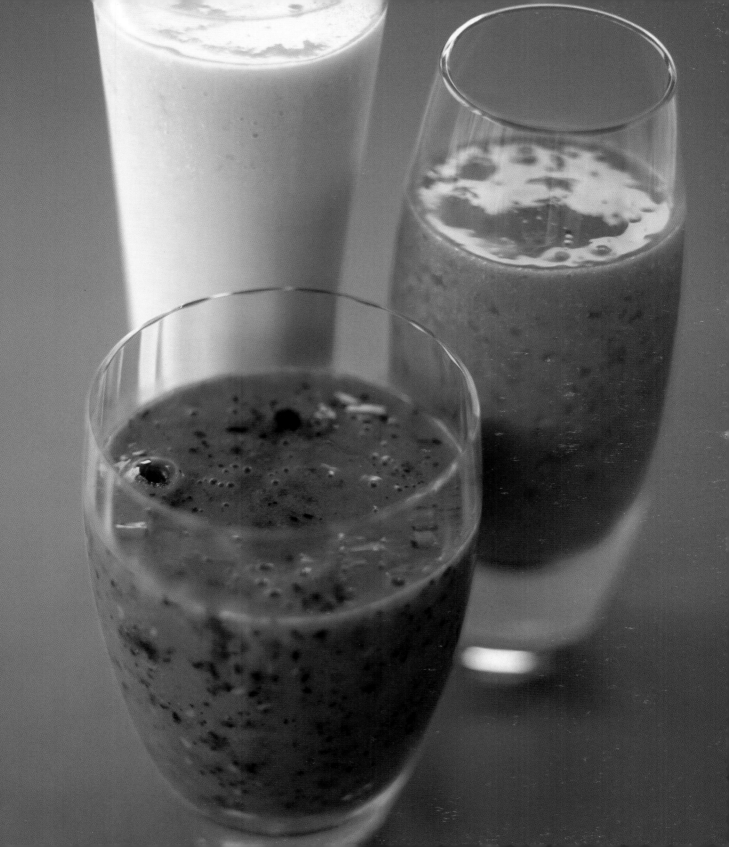

MANGO, APRICOT AND COCONUT SMOOTHIE

MAKES 2 DRINKS

1 mango, skinned, stone removed and chopped
4 ripe apricots, stoned and quartered
250 ml (8 fl oz) coconut milk
A few drops of vanilla extract
A cupful of crushed ice

▸ Place the ingredients in a smoothie maker, blender or food processor and blend until smooth and frothy. Serve immediately.

HEALTH STATISTICS
This drink packs a powerful antioxidant punch. It's bursting with beta-carotene, which improves immunity as well as helping promote smooth, healthy skin. Coconut milk is very low in fat.

NUTRITIONAL ANALYSIS (PER SERVING):

Calories 95 kcal	Carbohydrate 22 g
Protein 1.6 g	Total sugars* 22 g
Fat 0.6 g	Fibre 3.3 g
Saturates 0.3 g	Salt 0.3 g

* total sugars includes sugars found naturally in foods

BLUEBERRY BOOSTER

MAKES 2 DRINKS

125 g (4 oz) blueberries
250 ml (8 fl oz) apple juice
350 g (12 oz) blackberries
A handful of crushed ice

▸ Place the ingredients in a smoothie maker, blender or food processor and blend until smooth and frothy. Serve immediately.

HEALTH STATISTICS
Both blueberries and blackberries contain anthocyanins, extremely potent antioxidants that help guard against certain cancers, as well as benefiting your skin.

NUTRITIONAL ANALYSIS (PER SERVING):

Calories 107 kcal	Carbohydrate 24 g
Protein 2.3 g	Total sugars* 24 g
Fat 0.6 g	Fibre 7.4 g
Saturates 0.1 g	Salt 0.1 g

* total sugars includes sugars found naturally in foods

FOREST FRUITS CURE-ALL

MAKES 2 DRINKS

1 carton (150 g) cherry bio-yoghurt
200 ml (7 fl oz) cranberry juice drink
175 g (6 oz) frozen fruits-of-the-forest mixture, partially defrosted

▸ Combine the yoghurt and cranberry juice in a blender, smoothie maker or food processor. Add the fruits-of-the-forest mixture and blend until smooth.

HEALTH STATISTICS
Blueberries, cherries, strawberries and blackberries are all terrific sources of vitamin C and anthocyanins, antioxidants that bolster your immunity and protect against cancer.

NUTRITIONAL ANALYSIS (PER SERVING):

Calories 165 kcal	Carbohydrate 32 g
Protein 3.8 g	Total sugars* 32 g
Fat 2.4 g	Fibre 2.7 g
Saturates 1.5 g	Salt 0.1 g

* total sugars includes sugars found naturally in foods

PINEAPPLE AND GRAPEFRUIT SMOOTHIE

MAKES 2 DRINKS

2 rings fresh pineapple
Juice of 1 lime
Juice of ½ grapefruit
120 ml (4 fl oz) chilled water
1 teaspoon (5 ml) clear honey, to taste
A few ice cubes, to serve

▸ Place the pineapple, lime juice and grapefruit juice in a smoothie maker, blender or food processor and process until smooth. Add the water and honey and process until smooth. Pour into a glass, add a few ice cubes and serve immediately.

HEALTH STATISTICS
This delicious juice, packed with healing enzymes, will give you an energy boost. It's also rich in vitamin C.

NUTRITIONAL ANALYSIS (PER SERVING):

Calories 55 kcal	Carbohydrate 14 g
Protein 0.5 g	Total sugars* 14 g
Fat 0.2 g	Fibre 1.0 g
Saturates 0 g	Salt 0.1 g

* total sugars includes sugars found naturally in foods

PINEAPPLE AND ORANGE SMOOTHIE

MAKES 2 DRINKS

200 ml (7 fl oz) orange juice
125 g (4 oz) fresh pineapple, cut into pieces
1 banana, cut into chunks
6–8 ice cubes

▸ Place the ingredients in a smoothie maker, blender or food processor and blend until smooth and frothy. Serve immediately.

HEALTH STATISTICS
This smoothie provides good amounts of vitamin C from the orange juice and pineapple. The pineapple and banana both supply fibre and potassium, which is good for regulating fluid balance in the body.

NUTRITIONAL ANALYSIS (PER SERVING):

Calories 106 kcal	Carbohydrate 26 g
Protein 1.5 g	Total sugars* 25 g
Fat 0.3 g	Fibre 1.4 g
Saturates 0.1 g	Salt 0.1 g

* total sugars includes sugars found naturally in foods

APRICOT AND NECTARINE SMOOTHIE

MAKES 2 DRINKS

2 ripe nectarines, stoned and quartered
2 ripe apricots, stoned and quartered
125 ml (4 fl oz) orange juice
1 small banana, peeled and roughly chopped
About 10 ice cubes

▸ Place the ingredients in a smoothie maker, blender or food processor and blend until smooth and frothy. Serve immediately.

HEALTH STATISTICS
Rich in beta-carotene, fibre and vitamin C, this smoothie is great for promoting healthy smooth skin as well as protecting against cancer.

NUTRITIONAL ANALYSIS (PER SERVING):

Calories 141 kcal	Carbohydrate 33 g
Protein 3.4 g	Total sugars* 32 g
Fat 0.3 g	Fibre 3.1 g
Saturates 0.1 g	Salt 0.1 g

* total sugars includes sugars found naturally in foods

STRAWBERRY AND PAPAYA SMOOTHIE

MAKES 2 DRINKS

A small cupful of crushed ice
150 ml (5 fl oz) orange juice
125 g (4 oz) strawberries
$1/2$ papaya, peeled and roughly diced
$1/2$ banana

▸ Place the ingredients in a smoothie maker, blender or food processor and blend until smooth and frothy. Serve immediately.

HEALTH STATISTICS
Strawberries provide lots of immunity-boosting vitamin C while the papaya supplies beta-carotene, which helps promote healthy skin.

NUTRITIONAL ANALYSIS (PER SERVING):

Calories 93 kcal	Carbohydrate 22 g
Protein 1.5 g	Total sugars* 22 g
Fat 0.3 g	Fibre 2.6 g
Saturates 0.1 g	Salt 0.1 g

* total sugars includes sugars found naturally in foods

CAROL'S FAVOURITE PRODUCTS

To contact Carol e-mail: john@johnmiles.org.uk
Or Fax: 01275 810186

BOOKS

Detox For Life – the 28-Day plan
£10.99 First published 2001; revised edition 2002
This is the detox bible, a bestseller which has altered
the lives of thousands of people. Follow the detox plan
and weight loss and energy are guaranteed.

The Summer Detox 14-Day plan
£10.99 First published 2003; revised edition 2004
The summer detox was devised especially for those who
want to lose pounds to get into a new bikini. The recipes
use summer foods specifically so that you can benefit as
much as possible in a short space of time.

Detox Recipes
£11.99 First published 2003; revised edition 2005
This beautiful cookery book shows just how exciting and
tasty detox recipes can be. It includes dishes for the strict
detoxer and those on a maintenance plan and has proved
to be the ideal companion to the books above. This would
help anyone following the Cellulite 30-Day plan.

30-Day Cellulite Plan
£12.99 First published 2004
The original guide to combating cellulite, this book
contains full details on the causes of cellulite and a
comprehensive step-by-step 30-day plan to fight it,
accompanied by recipes, exercise and information
on creams and treatments.

SIMPLY ORGANIC 'IDEAL FOR DETOX' READY MEALS

In 2003 I tried a ready meal I'd bought in a supermarket
made by a small company called Simply Organic. It tasted
amazing, there were no additives and every ingredient
was organically grown. It was also very handy because,
as usual, I didn't have time to prepare a meal for one. As
a lot of detoxers need to take food to work with them or
have busy lives when they too don't have time to cook,
I thought it would be great to work with Simply Organic
to produce an 'Ideal For Detox' range. The range was
launched in late 2003 and is now available in most of the
big supermarkets in the UK. It includes soups and ready
meals and all of the range is suitable for anybody using
the Cellulite 30-Day plan.

Ideal For Detox Chunky Vegetable Soup
A really tasty veggie soup. Eat it alone, or with an
oatcake or rye bread.

Ideal for Detox Lentil and Parsley Soup
This soup is really thick and gorgeous and perfect for
autumn and winter days. It'll fill you up for the rest
of the day.

Ideal For Detox Mixed Bean Chilli
A wonderful chilli, there's a lot of it in the dish so if you
finish it, you're doing well. If you want to eat it in the
evening with brown rice and salad, even better. It's very
filling and you won't need any pudding afterwards.

Ideal For Detox Lentil and Winter Vegetable Stew
This dish is full of slow releasing energy. Eat it alone, or
with brown rice or rye bread.

Ideal For Detox Morroccan Vegetable Tagine
With a tangy tomato base this vegetable tagine is delicious

INDEX